THE SECRET TO
LOW CARB SUCCESS!

BOOK YOUR PLACE ON OUR WEBSITE AND MAKE THE READING CONNECTION!

We've created a customized website just for our very special readers, where you can get the inside scoop on everything that's going on with Zebra, Pinnacle and Kensington books.

When you come online, you'll have the exciting opportunity to:

- View covers of upcoming books
- Read sample chapters
- Learn about our future publishing schedule (listed by publication month *and author*)
- Find out when your favorite authors will be visiting a city near you
- Search for and order backlist books from our online catalog
- Check out author bios and background information
- Send e-mail to your favorite authors
- Meet the Kensington staff online
- Join us in weekly chats with authors, readers and other guests
- Get writing guidelines
- AND MUCH MORE!

**Visit our website at
http://www.kensingtonbooks.com**

The Secret to LOW CARB SUCCESS!

How to Get the Most Out of Your Low Carbohydrate Diet

LAURA RICHARD,
B.S.N., M.H.A.

KENSINGTON BOOKS
Kensington Publishing Corp.
http://www.kensingtonbooks.com

This book presents information based upon the research and personal experiences of the author. It is not intended to be a substitute for a professional consultation with a physician or other healthcare provider. Neither the publisher nor the author can be held responsible for any adverse effects or consequences resulting from the use of any of the information in this book. They also cannot be held responsible for any errors or omissions in this book. If you have a condition that requires medical advice, the publisher and author urge you to consult a competent healthcare professional.

KENSINGTON BOOKS are published by

Kensington Publishing Corp.
850 Third Avenue
New York, NY 10022

Copyright © 2001 by Laura Richard

All rights reserved. No part of this book may be reproduced in any form or by any means without the prior written consent of the Publisher, excepting brief quotes used in reviews.

If you purchased this book without a cover you should be aware that this book is stolen property. It was reported as "unsold and destroyed" to the Publisher and neither the Author nor the Publisher has received any payment for this "stripped book."

All Kensington Titles, Imprints, and Distributed Lines are available at special quantity discounts for bulk purchases for sales promotions, premiums, fund-raising, and educational or institutional use. Special book excerpts or customized printings can also be created to fit specific needs. For details, write or phone the office of the Kensington special sales manager: Kensington Publishing Corp., 850 Third Avenue, New York, NY 10022, attn: Special Sales Department, Phone: 1-800-221-2647.

Kensington and the K logo Reg. U.S. Pat. & TM Off.

First Printing: January 2002
10 9 8 7 6 5 4 3 2

Printed in the United States of America

To David, my best friend and husband.
To Jackie, who lights up every corner of my life.

Contents

Acknowledgments

Without my husband, David, this book would not exist. His willingness to spend long hours reading and editing the manuscript, often at the end of a day filled with work and child care, was a critical factor in my realizing my dream of writing this book. I will always appreciate his high-quality support and help.

Some of the others who helped me prepare this book are people I now consider to be among my newest friends. Special thanks go to editors Claire Gerus and Elaine Will Sparber for their expert advice and guidance in fully developing the manuscript. I also wish to thank Keith Sessions, who edited and polished the manuscript. He cheerfully assisted me on short notice to meet looming deadlines. Without these folks, this book would still only be a dream.

Introduction

Like many overweight people, I became intrigued with the "new revolution" of reduced carbohydrate dieting that has seized the attention of millions of dieters in the past few years. As a lifelong dieter, I had faithfully followed the advice of nutritional experts for most of my adult life. I ate a low fat diet made up of 60 to 75 percent carbohydrate, and I exercised. While I had some successes, they never lasted; I was constantly in a struggle to control my weight. Then, after the birth of my daughter, I found myself at my highest weight ever—and I was not happy about it. Even when my daughter turned three years old, I was still trying, with very little success, to lose the weight I had gained during my pregnancy.

Then I read some shocking statistics and information released by the National Institutes of Health (NIH) and Centers for Disease Control and Prevention (CDC). Obesity rates in the United States have become so high that the U.S. government routinely refers to obesity as an epidemic. In fact, obesity rates steadily rose through the 1990s until almost two-thirds (60 percent) of all Americans were overweight by 1999. The truly shocking aspect of these statistics is that our national weight continued to climb despite falling rates of fat consumption in the same period. I suddenly realized that I was not the only one who was faithfully following a low fat diet and not seeing any appreciable results. The whole country was having exactly the same experience I was! I came to a conclusion that I had really known all along: Low fat, high carbohydrate dieting was not working for me and I needed to look for another solution. I was *way* ready for a revolution.

So I began to research the alternatives. I read one of the books on low carbohydrate dieting. After that, I read another one. I read several books on reduced carbohydrate dieting, many of them multiple times. I was so persuaded by the theories in them that I started one of the diets despite the warnings of some nutritional experts. What I learned over the next several months was that reduced carbohydrate dieting truly is a revolution. I loved reduced carbohydrate dieting, and I loved the results I was getting. However, I also discovered that the diet was such a drastic change from my previous low fat eating style that I was learning a lot through trial and error—with an emphasis on the word "error." I was figuring it out, but it was taking a while. Then, after a few months on the diet, I realized that I was a slow loser compared to my family members and friends who had begun the diet at the same time. "What is going on here?" I thought. I was following all the rules faithfully, yet I was not losing weight as quickly as they were. After a while, I began to realize that I was very prone to slow weight loss and plateaus, and I began to have doubts. Maybe the critics are right and reduced carbohydrate dieting does not really work, I thought. Maybe it works for some people, but not for me. I was entertaining the notion of giving up. Had it not been for my husband's and family's ongoing success with the diet, I might have quit prematurely.

Instead of quitting, I decided to research reduced carbohydrate dieting on the Internet and learn more about it.

I began with the official web sites of the reduced carbohydrate diet experts. While I learned that periods of slow weight loss and plateaus are common in reduced carbohydrate dieting and that I should expect them, I did not get enough information about what to do about them. Then I got lucky and stumbled upon several great Internet support groups that offered advice and encouragement to new reduced carbohydrate dieters. The terrific feature of these message boards was that the advice was provided by reduced carbohydrate diet veterans, people who at one time had struggled with the diet as I was struggling. From this group of dedicated dieters, I learned all about the everyday aspects of living the reduced carbohydrate lifestyle that were not clearly or thoroughly covered in the books I had read. These dedicated dieters offered me information, support, and inspiration. They filled in the blanks for me, talked me through my doubts, and put me back on the path to weight loss. Although I remain one of the slower losers in these support groups, my rate of weight loss has sped up considerably by following their advice.

While I continued as a group participant for several months, I found that my role changed over time. I became one of the seasoned dieters offering advice to the "newbies." I loved passing on the information others had given me, plus sharing my personal insights. Through my active participation, I observed three trends that motivated me to write this book. First, there is a large volume of traffic on these enormously popular sites, with each site receiving hundreds, and some of them thousands, of visits each day from people seeking information about reduced carbohydrate dieting. I learned that I was not the only person who needed extra help. Second, I observed that a majority of the questions asked by the group participants were about how to speed weight loss, break weight loss stalls, and overcome plateaus. Last, I noticed that these questions were asked on the Internet message boards because they are not answered, or not answered clearly, in the currently available reduced carbohydrate diet books.

This handbook summarizes the wonderful, pragmatic, down-to-earth advice given by thousands of reduced carbohydrate diet veterans to newbies on how to speed weight loss and break through stalls and plateaus. It is not intended to explain the science of reduced carbohydrate dieting, but rather the mechanics of it. It is not intended to be a substitute for the popular reduced carbohydrate diet books written by the experts. Rather, it is meant to supplement these books by providing advice on how to live with the diet every day until it becomes second nature. This advice is valuable to the followers of a variety of reduced carbohydrate eating plans, whether ketogenic or nonketogenic.

My experience and the experiences of others have taught me that it takes a while for someone to really learn how to be successful on a reduced carbohydrate diet. The factors that lead to success and the problems that hinder it are highly individualized. Because we all react somewhat differently to reduced carbohydrate dieting, there is a period of experimentation that we all must go through to learn the factors that stall our weight loss and the factors that speed it up again. This process can take several weeks or months, depending upon the individual; but for all of us, it takes time. It takes so much time and effort because reduced carbohydrate dieting is a complete reversal from the low fat dieting that we practiced for years, and it is not well supported in our sugar-laden world. While acceptance of the diet has improved, we reduced carbohydrate dieters, especially the new ones, still find that we are no longer in the cultural mainstream of eating and must learn to find our own way.

One of the things that struck me a few weeks into reduced carbohydrate dieting was that proof of our society's strong addiction to carbohydrate is ever-present in our everyday language. For example, a lucrative business deal is a "sweet deal." Our lovers are our "sweethearts," and if we are lucky, they whisper "sweet nothings" in our ears before we drift off to sleep to have "sweet dreams." An extra benefit is called "icing on the cake," something easy is referred to as "gravy," and our aspirations are "pie in the sky." The list is endless and can be a source of amusement for reduced carbohydrate dieters.

In addition to overcoming our society's addiction to carbohydrate, we reduced carbohydrate dieters must completely rid ourselves of the most cherished assumptions taught to us over the years by "nutritional experts" who advocate low fat, high carbohydrate dieting. For example, many of us previously eliminated low carbohydrate foods from our menus in an effort to lower our fat intake. Now we must learn to once again cook with them. We may find that restaurants that were once our favorites no longer have an attraction for us as we discover the menus are not hospitable to our new reduced carbohydrate diet. On the other hand, restaurants we would not have considered patronizing in our low fat dieting days are now havens for us.

The challenge for new reduced carbohydrate dieters is to establish an approach to eating that allows weight loss in a world in which sugar is highly valued by all. The goal of this book is to support you in quickly developing the required skills that will allow you to succeed. My hope is that you will work through the trial and error stage more quickly and easily by learning from the experiences of others. My aim is to assist you in understanding slow weight loss, stalls, and plateaus, including their common causes and the actions that reverse them. Most of all, my goal is to provide you with support as you make your way in our high carbohydrate world. I am confident that this advice, along with a healthy dose of patience and persistence, will put you on track for a satisfying rate of weight loss.

First, we need a basic understanding of the variety of reduced carbohydrate diet books on the market. The first chapter of this book provides summaries of the most popular reduced carbohydrate dieting plans. They range from low carbohydrate plans, such as *Dr. Atkins' New Diet Revolution* and *Protein Power*, to mid-range plans, such as *The Zone* and *Sugar Busters!* (For the publishing data for all the reduced carbohydrate diet books discussed in this book, see Chapter 6.) The second chapter discusses what to expect when you embark on a reduced carbohydrate diet. It includes information on how much you can expect to lose and how quickly you can expect to lose it, the common patterns of weight loss, and how muscle growth masks fat loss. The next two chapters, Chapters 3 and 4, give specific information about the factors widely believed to slow weight loss and cause plateaus, and what to do about them. Chapter 5 summarizes the reduced carbohydrate diet book authors' advice about maximizing success as presented in their books and on their web sites. And finally, Chapter 6 offers a wealth of resources for reduced carbohydrate dieters, including an extensive list of relevant books, cookbooks, discussion groups, web sites, and newsletters.

A word of caution: While the greatest benefit of advice given by seasoned reduced carbohydrate dieters is that it is from people who have "been there and done that," it is not from medical experts. The advice presented in this handbook is for informational purposes only and should not be interpreted as medical advice. It should not be taken as a substitute for medical consultation, and all readers are strongly encouraged to consult their personal physicians. No claims of therapeutic benefits for the treatment of any illness or disability are made. The Food and Drug Administration (FDA) has not evaluated the information in this book.

The examples given in this book are stories derived from the Internet support groups that I visit frequently. All the names have been changed, and some examples are compilations of the experiences of multiple persons. These stories have been combined for illustrative purposes and in the interests of brevity and clarity.

With that said, let's move on to the diets, whooshes, Carbo Witch, stalls, and plateaus, and learn how you can become a successful low carbohydrate dieter!

1
The Diets in a Nutshell

Before we jump into a discussion of the pesky stumbling blocks that can lead to irritating periods of slow weight loss, stalls, and plateaus, it is important that we explore the various reduced carbohydrate diet plans and gain a basic understanding of the theories behind them and the similarities and differences among them. Because this book is not specific to any single reduced carbohydrate diet plan, it is important that we look at all the major reduced carbohydrate diet books, the theories that form their basis, and the authors' views on how best to use reduced carbohydrate dieting to our advantage. Although these authors have differences of opinion that, in effect, provide us with a cornucopia of choices, there are several aspects of reduced carbohydrate dieting upon which they all agree. Let's begin our discussion with these points of agreement.

Points of Agreement

Given the ferocity of the debate about reduced carbohydrate dieting that is raging among medical and nutritional professionals (and that occasionally infiltrates even the ranks of the reduced carbohydrate diet experts themselves), we might incorrectly assume that there are no points of agreement among the professionals when it comes to reduced carbohydrate dieting. However, as research in the area of reduced carbohydrate dieting becomes more refined and part of the mainstream in medical literature, several major theories have developed upon which all the reduced carbohydrate diet book authors agree.

Excess Carbohydrate Is the Problem

Basically, all the reduced carbohydrate diet book authors agree that too much carbohydrate, particularly too much simple, refined carbohydrate, is the fundamental cause of obesity. They believe that too much carbohydrate in our diets leads us to overproduce insulin, which in turn leads to an overcreation of body fat. This fundamental concept is the common characteristic that groups all of these plans together and the factor that sets them apart from low calorie and low fat diets.

Here is a simple explanation of the underlying theory upon which they all agree. Our bodies use three basic macronutrients for energy: carbohydrate, protein, and fat. While our bodies have the ability to convert all three of these to blood glucose, fat and protein are converted slowly while carbohydrate is converted quickly. Therefore, protein and fat cause small, slow rises in the blood glucose levels (fat the slowest and smallest of all), while carbohydrate causes large, rapid rises.

Our bodies produce a hormone in the pancreas known as insulin. Insulin's job is to lower the level of glucose in our blood by triggering several important biological processes that move the glucose into our cells so the cells can use it for energy. If we have more glucose in our blood than our cells need, insulin acts further by prompting our livers to store the excess glucose in a temporary form known as glycogen. (Glycogen is stored in our liver and other body tissues, such as muscle, from which it can be easily pulled as a quick source of energy.) Once our bodies have enough glycogen in store, insulin triggers biological processes that prompt our livers to convert any excess glucose to a more permanent form of storage—it becomes body fat.

Obviously, insulin plays several critical roles in our survival. First, it helps our cells to get the glucose they need to power critical biological functions. Second, it keeps our blood sugar levels within a normal range, which is important because prolonged periods of excess blood glucose can have several serious detrimental effects on our bodies. Third, it aids in the storage of body fat, which is important for survival during periods of famine (not a problem for us lately, but critical nonetheless).

Therefore, when we eat carbohydrate, our blood glucose levels rise and insulin is released in response. The amount of insulin released is directly proportional to how much and how quickly our blood sugar levels rise. If our blood glucose rises quickly and/or reaches high levels, large amounts of insulin are released. If our blood glucose levels rise slowly and/or peak at low to moderate levels, little insulin is released. *The key mechanism that we must clearly understand is that the greater the amount of carbohydrate we eat, the greater the amount of insulin we produce and the greater the amount of body fat we create.* Our primary goal, therefore, is to control the amount of insulin we produce by controlling the amount of carbohydrate we eat. The less carbohydrate we eat, the less insulin we produce and the less body fat we store.

For most people, this carbohydrate–insulin–body fat storage cycle is in balance, as nature intended it to be. We all know these folks: They eat whatever they want and gain little to no weight. (While some of these people can be quite the nuisance to those of us struggling with our weight, since our nation's carbohydrate intake has risen over the past 20 years, they are becoming harder and harder to find.)

Then there are the rest of us. We are the unfortunate souls who do not have balanced carbohydrate–insulin–body fat storage cycles, but instead are caught in vicious cycles of weight gain. When we eat too much carbohydrate, our blood sugar levels rise very quickly and/or very high. Our pancreas overreacts and swiftly releases large amounts of insulin in response, often much more insulin than is necessary to do the job. The insulin triggers the normal biological processes that offer the glucose to our cells to be used for energy. However, if our cells say, in essence, "No thanks, we're full," or if they are unable to accept the glucose (as is the case in insulin resistance, discussed later) the insulin triggers the other biological processes that allow the blood glucose to be stored as glycogen and body fat.

The problem for many of us is that insulin does its job only too well. When we produce too much insulin, too much glucose is removed from our blood, too much body fat is created, our blood glucose levels plunge, and we become hungry again. (When our blood glucose levels fall too low, it is known as hypoglycemia, with the prefix *hypo* meaning "too little," *gly* referring to glucose, and *cemia* meaning "in the blood.") This process can occur very quickly, and we can find that we have symptoms of low blood sugar (including hunger) in only one to three hours after we ate the carbohydrate. In fact, this symptom is the hallmark of all the symptoms that indicate we have a problem in properly handling carbohydrate: Although we eat substantial amounts of food, when it is made up of carbohydrate, we are hungry again within a few short hours. This hunger prompts us to crave and eat more carbohydrate, and the cycle begins all over again.

For those of us caught in this destructive cycle, it feels as though we are in a constant battle to control our hunger. The reduced carbohydrate diet book authors say that we must learn we cannot control our hunger and weight by eating high amounts of carbohydrate. In fact, eating too much carbohydrate does not slay the dragon—it feeds and strengthens it. It is analogous to attempting to put out a fire by pouring gasoline on it.

For those of us with this problem, carbohydrate causes us to be hungry nearly continuously. If we respond to the hunger by eating more carbohydrate, we give our bodies a continuous supply of glucose. Our bodies respond by producing a continuous supply of insulin. (This continuous presence of insulin is known as hyperinsulinemia, with the prefix *hyper* meaning "too much", and *emia* meaning "in the blood.") This oversupply of insulin completes the vicious cycle by creating too much body fat. This theory explains why we are constantly hungry even while we are gaining weight. The solution, according to the reduced carbohydrate diet experts, is to break the cycle by reducing our carbohydrate intake.

Insulin Resistance May Be a Problem

For some of us, the problem is not an overproduction of insulin, but rather our cells not reacting to insulin properly. This condition, known as insulin resistance, occurs when the cells become resistant to the effects of insulin.

As we just discussed, one of the jobs of insulin is to move glucose from the blood into our cells so the cells can use it for energy. When the cells resist the action of insulin, the glucose cannot enter the cells and it remains in the blood. As a result, the cells lack the energy they need to function, and they send out hunger signals. This phenomenon explains why people who have insulin resistance can have chronically elevated blood glucose levels, high insulin levels, chronic hunger, and weight gain simultaneously. Because the cells cannot accept the glucose, the liver converts the glucose left stranded in the blood to body fat.

Insulin May Have Other Negative Effects

The reduced carbohydrate diet book authors also agree that prolonged excessive insulin levels can lead not only to obesity, but to several other serious illnesses as well. In fact, most of the authors believe that many of the major chronic illnesses of our day are directly related to elevated insulin levels. The illnesses they collectively mention are diabetes, insulin resistance, hypoglycemia, heart disease, excess fluid retention, hypertension, atherosclerosis (hardening of the arteries), high cholesterol, poor cholesterol ratios, high triglycerides, depression, alcoholism, chronic fatigue syndrome, premenstrual syndrome, and some forms of cancer. They say that hyperinsulinemia is the common link that explains why these diseases are more prevalent among the obese. The hyperinsulinemia that causes their excess body fat is the very factor that places overweight people at risk for these chronic illnesses.

Glucagon Suppression Leads to Weight Gain

The reduced carbohydrate diet book authors also agree that another major effect of excessive carbohydrate intake is that it suppresses the production of glucagon. Glucagon is the hormone produced by the pancreas that has the opposite function of insulin when it comes to regulating body fat stores. While insulin triggers the processes that cause blood glucose to be converted to body fat, glucagon triggers the processes that cause body fat to be converted back to blood glucose—our ultimate goal. Therefore, our bodies must produce and release glucagon to break down body fat. Unfortunately, our pancreas will not release glucagon, or will release it only in small amounts, if we have continuously high levels of glucose and insulin in our blood. Look at it this way: If you continuously have a level of cash flowing into your household that is high enough to meet all of your expenses (and then some), why would you go to the bank to withdraw funds from your savings? It is much the same with glucagon. A rich flow of carbohydrate in our blood blocks us from dipping into our body fat stores ("savings") for energy. Therefore, in those of us who are caught in this unhealthy cycle that produces high levels of insulin, glucagon is rarely released and, as a result, we do not lose weight.

The absence of glucagon also affects our health in many ways. The beneficial effects of glucagon are allowing our kidneys to release fluid and thereby reducing fluid retention, telling our cardiovascular and nervous systems to lower our blood pressure, and signaling our livers to lower our triglyceride and cholesterol levels.

It is important to note that while Dr. Atkins agrees with this basic principle, he believes that instead of glucagon, a hormone produced by the pituitary gland known as a fat mobilizing hormone is what breaks down fat. However, he does agree that the presence of glucose and insulin in the bloodstream inhibits the release of the hormone and, therefore, hinders the fat breakdown.

Reduced Carbohydrate Is the Key to Success

It should be obvious by now that all the authors agree that the only way to break the cycle and correct the underlying problem of too much insulin and not enough glucagon is to control the amount of carbohydrate we eat. They believe that less carbohydrate in our diets leads to lower blood glucose levels, which in turn lead to less insulin production and more glucagon production. Therefore, less carbohydrate in our diets allows our bodies to minimize how much blood glucose is stored as body fat.

The Calorie Theory Does Not Work

All of the authors agree that using the calorie theory for weight loss is not effective. Their basic criticism of the calorie theory is that simply counting calories does not take into account the fact that each of the macronutrients has a different effect on our bodies. Carbohydrate causes sharp and rapid increases in our blood glucose levels, while protein causes slow and steady increases in our blood glucose levels and fat causes little or no increases in our blood glucose levels. Therefore, 100 calories of carbohydrate cause greater insulin release than do 100 calories of protein, and 100 calories of fat cause the least amount of insulin release of all. According to these authors, 100 calories of carbohydrate have far more "fattening power" than 100 calories of the other two macronutrients. The calorie theory is faulty, they say, because it does not take these differences into account.

While all the authors agree the calorie theory is not valid as a basis for losing weight, they do agree that too much food leads to slow weight loss. Several of them—Dr. Sears (*The Zone*), Dr. Pescatore (*Thin for Good*), and the authors of *Sugar Busters!*—recommend portion control as part of their plan. The remaining authors differ in that they do not believe we should restrict the amount of food we eat unless we are having a great deal of difficulty losing weight or are stuck in plateaus. This topic is covered more fully in Chapter 3.

Low Fat Diets Do Not Work

Because these authors strongly agree that too much insulin is the root cause of obesity, they also agree that low fat diets not only fail to work, but actually aggravate the underlying problem. As stated above, they believe that of all the macronutrients, fat causes the least amount of insulin to be produced. Therefore, restricting dietary fat and replacing it with carbohydrate causes higher insulin levels and adds body fat. Omitting fat from the diet also sacrifices taste and satiety; we are less satisfied with the food we eat. Carbohydrate does not stay with us as long as fat does. Therefore, we are hungry more and satisfied less. (It should be noted that while all of these authors agree that low fat diets are ineffective as a basis for losing weight, they vary widely on how much and what types of fat should be included in our diet.)

Exercise Works

All the authors agree that exercise is a critical component of weight loss, and most of them recommend moderate exercise and strength training (weight lifting).

Points of Difference

Although all these authors fundamentally agree that carbohydrate intake must be cut to lose weight, they differ on how much it should be reduced. On one end of the spectrum, some of them advocate very low levels of carbohydrate and significant amounts of protein and fat because they believe it is most beneficial to produce little or no insulin while producing large amounts of glucagon. On the other end of the spectrum, other reduced carbohydrate diet experts believe that small amounts of insulin are beneficial for dieters and necessary for overall health. They suggest a diet with a balance of carbohydrate and protein to balance insulin and glucagon releases.

The degree to which the reduced carbohydrate diet book authors recommend restricting carbohydrate is not their only point of difference. While these contradictions can be confusing, the good news is that a full range of options is available to us through these various plans. Many successful reduced carbohydrate dieters have put together their own unique approach by borrowing concepts from each of the authors. You may wish to do the same. To guide you in your choices, following are the major points upon which the reduced carbohydrate diet book authors differ.

Ketosis

One of the major differences among the reduced carbohydrate diet experts is whether or not ketosis is a safe method for losing weight. Ketosis is a state of rapid body fat breakdown that occurs when carbohydrate is restricted to very low levels, usually 30 to 40 grams per day. The theory is that ketosis occurs when the body releases large amounts of glucagon, depleting its readily available stores of glucose (namely, the glucose in the blood and all the available supplies of glycogen), and turns nearly exclusively to body fat stores for energy. When body fat is broken down rapidly, small fragments known as ketone bodies are produced. These ketone bodies enter the bloodstream and are used by the cells as fuel. When this process occurs, a person is said to be in a state of ketosis. Diets that induce ketosis are known as ketogenic diets, with *keto* referring to the process of ketosis and *genic* meaning "the creation of."

Two of today's popular low carbohydrate diets, *Dr. Atkins' New Diet Revolution* and *Protein Power*, are ketogenic; they restrict carbohydrate intake to the point that ketosis results. The authors of these two diet plans strongly believe that ketosis is a valuable tool in losing body fat. They believe ketosis is a safe, natural process that allows rapid breakdown of body fat while maintaining beneficial lean body mass.

However, other reduced carbohydrate diet experts feel equally strongly that ketosis should be avoided. They believe that ketosis is an emergency measure taken by the body as a last-ditch effort to prevent starvation and that it places the body under unnecessary stress. In particular, Dr. Sears states in *The Zone* that he believes ketone bodies are fragments resulting from the breakdown of body protein and other lean body tissues, not body fat stores. Therefore, Dr. Sears and others differ from Dr. Atkins and the authors of *Protein Power* in that they do not recommend carbohydrate intake be restricted to the point of inducing ketosis.

The Glycemic Index

Several of the reduced carbohydrate diet book authors refer to the glycemic index, a rating system that ranks the effects of individual foods on the level of glucose in the blood. Originally developed in the early 1980s to guide diabetics in their food choices, the glycemic index is also helpful for those of us who are on reduced carbohydrate diets. Foods that have rapid and marked effects on our blood glucose levels are said to have high glycemic index values. These foods are generally considered to be undesirable sources of carbohydrate because they cause our blood glucose to rise quickly to high levels and, therefore, the pancreas to release large amounts of insulin. Examples of foods with high glycemic index values are refined white bread, table sugar, pasta, and potatoes.

On the other hand, some foods have a slower and less striking impact on our blood glucose levels. These foods are said to have low glycemic index values. Low glycemic index foods are generally considered to be more desirable because they are digested more slowly. They cause our blood glucose levels to rise more slowly and, therefore, the pancreas to produce less insulin in response. Generally, low glycemic index foods include high fiber, unprocessed, "natural" foods such as whole, fresh vegetables.

The degree to which the reduced carbohydrate diet experts advocate using the glycemic index to guide food choices varies widely. On one end of the spectrum are the *Sugar Busters!* authors, who strongly advocate using the glycemic index. In fact, one of the authors refers to the glycemic index as the "foundation of the diet." On the other end of the spectrum are the *Protein Power* authors, who discourage the use of the glycemic index and instead offer an alternative method of using fiber count to estimate the impact of foods on blood glucose levels. This method is known as the effective carbohydrate count. Both the glycemic index and the effective carbohydrate count are discussed in Chapter 4 of this book.

Which Diet Is Right for You?

As you will see when you read the following summaries of the most popular reduced carbohydrate diet plans, the underlying theories of why and how high carbohydrate diets lead to obesity are basically the same, but the recommended approaches for correcting the problem are quite different. The degree of success and satisfaction you will experience on any one of these plans has a great deal to do with your personality, preferences, and health goals. Which plan is attractive to you may very well be contingent on the following factors, among others:

- How much weight you wish to lose
- How quickly you wish to lose it
- How much structure you want in your diet
- The amount of carbohydrate restriction you can tolerate
- Your beliefs about the health benefits of each plan
- Your degree of carbohydrate addiction
- Your overall goals, such as weight loss or disease reversal
- Your beliefs about the safety and effectiveness of ketosis

To help you determine which of these plans fits best with your lifestyle and preferences, this chapter includes brief summaries of the most popular reduced carbohydrate diet plans. But first, a couple of notes about the summaries: They focus specifically on weight loss, although several authors include in their books information about the benefits of reduced carbohydrate dieting in improving overall health and resolving chronic illnesses. Second, each summary includes a brief overview of the plan, a review of the book, and some information on why the followers of the plan say they like it. Third, the summaries are not intended to be replacements for reading the actual books. They are just meant to give you an idea of the general principles of the diets to help you choose which of the books you would like to read in their entirety. Fourth, the books are listed in the order in which they were published to give you an idea of how the reduced carbohydrate diet movement evolved. And last, the authors' advice with respect to slow weight loss and plateaus is presented in Chapter 5.

For a quick review of the information presented in the summaries and an at-a-glance comparison of the diets, see Table 1.1 on page 99.

Dr. Atkins' New Diet Revolution

Dr. Robert C. Atkins is widely regarded as the founding father of modern reduced carbohydrate dieting. He is a practicing cardiologist who founded and continues to practice at the Atkins Center for Complementary Medicine in New York City. He claims a remarkable record; he states on his web site that he has successfully treated 60,000 people with low carbohydrate dieting and nutritional supplementation. Of these 60,000 patients, approximately 25,000 were treated for weight problems and 35,000 were treated for a variety of conditions including heart disease, hypertension, diabetes, and hypoglycemia.

Dr. Atkins' first book, *Dr. Atkins' Diet Revolution*, was originally published in 1972. It caused a huge sensation in the world of dieting, but in the 1980s, low fat dieting became the method preferred by nutritional experts and professional medical organizations such as the American Heart Association and the American Diabetes Association. All the low carbohydrate diets of the day, including Dr. Atkins' diet, fell from favor.

In 1992, Dr. Atkins' second book was released, under the title of *Dr. Atkins' New Diet Revolution*. The same as its predecessor, it became a tremendous sensation, and it caused a second dieting "revolution." In 1997, the book became a bestseller, and it has remained on *The New York Times* best-seller list for over four years. An updated and revised version of this book was released in 1999. The phenomenal sales of Dr. Atkins' second book fueled another firestorm of controversy among nutritional experts and the medical community, primarily because it strongly recommends ketosis as the preferred method for reducing body fat.

The Plan

Dr. Atkins' diet is perhaps the most straightforward of all the reduced carbohydrate plans. In the updated 1999 version of his book, *Dr. Atkins' New Diet Revolution*, Dr. Atkins presents the three basic tenets of his approach. The first is the restriction of carbohydrate to very low levels, usually less than 40 grams per day; the second is nutritional supplementation; and the third is exercise.

The foundation of Dr. Atkins' diet is the thesis that nearly all obesity is a direct result of metabolic disturbances, not overeating. In fact, he asserts that many overweight people eat fewer calories than people who do not have weight problems. If a person is seriously overweight or has been overweight for an extended period, Dr. Atkins believes it is almost always a result of disturbed carbohydrate metabolism and excess insulin production. He divides people who have this metabolic disturbance into three distinct groups.

The first group consists of people who are naturally resistant to losing weight or who have difficulty achieving satiety because of basic metabolic problems. The second group is made up of people with hypoglycemia. And the third group consists of people with carbohydrate addiction. Dr. Atkins views his diet as a corrective diet that rectifies all three of these problems through carbohydrate restriction. He believes that limiting carbohydrate intake interrupts the destructive cycle that causes excessive insulin production and weight gain.

Ketosis

Dr. Atkins recommends restricting carbohydrate intake to the point at which insulin is not released or is released in very small amounts. Dr. Atkins' diet is ketogenic, meaning it restricts carbohydrate to the extent that the body goes into a state he calls Benign Dietary Ketosis, commonly referred to as ketosis. Dr. Atkins asserts that ketone bodies are natural, beneficial byproducts of the breakdown of stored body fat.

According to Dr. Atkins, ketosis occurs for most people when carbohydrate intake is restricted to 40 grams or less per day. However, he says that 40 percent of metabolically resistant women must reduce their carbohydrate intake to 30 grams or less per day for fat loss to occur. Dr. Atkins advises dieters that to keep losing weight, they must continue this degree of carbohydrate restriction. If they ingest carbohydrate, their bodies will use the carbohydrate as fuel and the state of ketosis will end.

Dr. Atkins strongly recommends ketosis as the preferred method for losing weight, and he is not supportive of reduced carbohydrate diets that do not induce it. In his opinion, the amount of weight lost is directly proportional to the degree to which carbohydrate intake is restricted. Without significant reductions in carbohydrate intake, significant weight loss will not occur quickly. He states that ketosis is a safe, natural process, and he refers to it as a metabolic advantage. He considers it advantageous because it enables dieters to eat many more calories than on other diets and still lose body fat. He advocates a ketogenic diet because he believes that ketosis is the process in which fat is broken down at the fastest rate, and it has the added benefits of depressing the appetite and sparing lean body mass. Dr. Atkins believes that dieters are at an unnecessary disadvantage without ketosis.

Pre-Diet Preparations

Dr. Atkins recommends that dieters get a medical checkup, including a glucose tolerance test, to establish their overall health, cholesterol levels, triglyceride level, glucose level, insulin level, and thyroid function before beginning the diet. He states that this information is useful in demonstrating the success of the diet later. He also recommends that dieters consult their physicians about discontinuing any unnecessary medications, herbs, and dietary supplements. He also recommends that dieters consult their physicians about adjusting the dosage of any diuretics or diabetes medications they may be taking. Ketogenic diets are naturally diuretic. Therefore, less diuretic medication is usually required. Likewise, lower glucose levels occur when the amount of ingested carbohydrate is reduced. Therefore, less diabetic medication is usually required.

Four Phases

Dr. Atkins recommends that his diet be undertaken in four phases. In all four phases, simple carbohydrate sources such as sugar, white flour, pasta, milk, and white rice are not allowed. In each phase, the amount of complex, or "healthy," carbohydrate is progressively increased. The first phase, which is the most carbohydrate restrictive, is known as the Induction diet and lasts for 14 days. In this phase, all dieters are restricted to 20 grams of carbohydrate or less per day. The goal of the induction phase is to quickly break carbohydrate addiction and interrupt the destructive cycle of excessive insulin production by inducing ketosis quickly (usually within 48 hours).

The second phase is known as the Ongoing Weight Loss (OWL) diet. It begins on the fifteenth day and continues until the goal weight is reached. In this phase, dieters are instructed to raise their daily intake of complex carbohydrate in 5-gram increments until they reach the point where weight loss stops. Dr. Atkins calls the point at which weight loss stops the Critical Carbohydrate Level for Losing (CCLL). This point is the maximum amount of carbohydrate dieters can consume and still continue to lose weight. Eating carbohydrate above this level causes weight loss to stop, while eating below this level allows weight loss to continue. The point at which this occurs is specific to each dieter. (Dr. Atkins also says in his book that dieters may voluntarily remain at or below 20 grams of carbohydrate per day for as long as they feel good as an alternative to raising their intake.)

The third phase is known as the Pre-Maintenance diet, and it begins when the goal weight is in sight. The goal of the Pre-Maintenance diet is to transition from the weight loss phase to the "real world" of lifetime weight maintenance. Dr. Atkins recommends that dieters slow their weight loss to the point at which the last 5 to 10 pounds are lost at a rate of about 1 pound per week. The idea is to gradually increase the carbohydrate count to slow down weight loss in preparation for the last phase, known as the Maintenance diet.

The Maintenance diet is the phase in which dieters eat for the remainder of their life. Dr. Atkins believes that people who have difficulty appropriately processing carbohydrate will be challenged with this metabolic disturbance throughout their lives and, therefore, must restrict carbohydrate accordingly. In this phase, dieters establish a second carbohydrate level, which Dr. Atkins calls the Critical Carbohydrate Level for Maintenance (CCLM). This level of carbohydrate is the maximum amount dieters can ingest without regaining weight. Dr. Atkins says most people reach their CCLM at somewhere between 40 and 60 grams of carbohydrate per day. By definition, eating carbohydrate at or below the CCLM allows dieters to maintain their new low weight, while eating above it causes them to gain weight.

Even in the maintenance phase, Dr. Atkins strongly discourages eating simple and refined carbohydrate. He instructs dieters to derive their carbohydrate intake from vegetables, whole grains, and some low sugar fruits. He cautions dieters that reintroducing unhealthy refined sugars will serve only to reactivate the metabolic disturbances that caused their original weight gain. He warns dieters that they will never be "cured" of the underlying metabolic disturbance; his diet will simply get around it.

Dr. Atkins mentions two basic pitfalls that cause dieters to gain weight during the maintenance phase. First, many people find they must learn new skills to keep their carbohydrate count low without the appetite-suppressing effects of ketosis. And second, dieters are often surprised at how narrow the range of carbohydrate intake can be before weight gain recurs. Dr. Atkins advises dieters that any weight gain of 5 pounds or more should be immediately handled by returning to the induction phase. He advises that ketosis be induced and maintained until the weight has once again been lost.

Fat

Dr. Atkins does not support the medical community's recommendation to restrict dietary fat. He lists several benefits of dietary fat, and he cautions people against doing a low fat version of his diet. He promotes dietary fat because he says it satisfies the appetite, stabilizes the blood sugar, and stops carbohydrate cravings. According to Dr. Atkins, the greatest benefit of dietary fat is that in the absence of carbohydrate, it increases the rate at which stored fat is burned. He counters the medical criticism of this belief by saying that because of the satiety caused by fat, many of his patients eat *less* fat than they did before beginning his diet.

Dr. Atkins does not differentiate between the benefits or drawbacks of the various sources of fat in his book. He does caution dieters against eating trans fat. He believes that, with the exception of trans fat, dietary fat does not cause heart disease.

Fiber

Dr. Atkins does not give his opinion of the glycemic index in *Dr. Atkins' New Diet Revolution,* but he supports it in a later book, *Dr. Atkins' Age-Defying Diet Revolution.* In his original books printed in 1972 and 1992, Dr. Atkins does not mention the practice of subtracting the fiber count from the carbohydrate count, thereby including in the daily carbohydrate count only the carbohydrate that can be digested. However, in the updated 1999 version of *Dr. Atkins' New Diet Revolution,* he supports the practice. (For futher discussions of this practice, see Chapter 4 of this book.)

Nutritional Supplements

Dr. Atkins is a strong believer in the benefits of nutritional supplementation in all phases of his diet. He recommends nutritional supplementation not only for weight loss, but also for overall health. He believes strongly in treating many medical conditions with nutrients rather than with conventional drugs and medicine, and he sees weight loss as no exception.

Dr. Atkins asserts that there are three primary reasons nutritional supplements are important for low carbohydrate dieters. Many dieters who were previously on low fat diets are likely to be deficient in the essential fatty acids and fat-soluble vitamins. Likewise, dieters who previously consumed large amounts of high carbohydrate junk food are likely to be deficient in several other critical nutrients. And lastly, a number of nutrients are important in maximizing the body's ability to burn fat, especially among people who have difficulty losing weight. (This topic is covered in detail in Chapter 4 of this book.)

Exercise

The third tenet of Dr. Atkins' program concerns exercise. Dr. Atkins strongly advocates exercise in addition to carbohydrate restriction, especially for people who find it difficult to lose weight. He refers to exercise as "tremendously important" and believes that it reduces the production of insulin.

About the Book

For many people, the biggest attraction of *Dr. Atkins' New Diet Revolution* is its relative simplicity as compared to the other reduced carbohydrate diet books. Dr. Atkins presents his theories of why and how low carbohydrate diets work in a straightforward, uncomplicated fashion, and this may explain in part why the book is the most popular of all the reduced carbohydrate diet books. For the most part, the book does not contain a great deal of complicated science and biology. It is a great primer for people who want to understand the basic theories of how and why low carbohydrate dieting works, but do not wish to delve too deeply into the scientific detail.

For the most part, *Dr. Atkins' New Diet Revolution* is a focused book; it has a strong concentration on the topic of losing weight. Although he briefly discusses the positive effects of low carbohydrate dieting on other illnesses, such as hypertension and heart disease, he saves the detailed discussions of these benefits for other books. Those people who are embarking on low carbohydrate dieting primarily for weight loss can readily find the information they need without having to sort through a lot of other information.

Dr. Atkins' New Diet Revolution contains more information about slow weight loss, stalls, and plateaus than do the other reduced carbohydrate diet books. Dr. Atkins spends a significant amount of time addressing the issue that some people lose weight at much slower rates than do others. He uses the term "metabolic resistance" to address these variations, and he devotes an entire chapter to the topic of extreme metabolic resistance.

Dr. Atkins is quite passionate about low carbohydrate dieting, and his passion is evident throughout the book. A significant portion of the book is devoted to countering the criticisms of his diet leveled by the medical community. People who are seeking a good understanding of the medical controversy surrounding Dr. Atkins' diet and his responses to them find this book to be very helpful in clarifying the controversy.

The book contains menus and recipes appropriate for the Induction, Ongoing Weight Loss, Pre-Maintenance, and Maintenance phases of the diet. It also includes a carbohydrate gram counter and an extensive bibliography.

Why Followers Like the Diet

Judging by the degree of activity of Dr. Atkins' supporters on the Internet and the volume of sales of *Dr. Atkins' New Diet Revolution*, it appears that the Atkins diet is the most popular of the reduced carbohydrate diet plans. In the Internet support groups and on the discussion boards, the Atkins diet is by far the diet discussed most often. Of the message boards devoted to a single diet plan, the Atkins message boards are the most numerous and the most active. The followers of the Atkins diet tend to be quite loyal, and many affectionately refer to themselves as Atkids. Like Dr. Atkins, they have a passion for low carbohydrate dieting in general and the Atkins diet in particular.

The general consensus among Atkins diet followers is that simplicity is the greatest strength of the plan. Basically, dieters need only find the maximum amount of carbohydrate they can eat each day and still maintain ketosis, and lose weight until they reach their goal weights. The plan does not call for weighing, measuring, or tracking food intake other than counting grams of carbohydrate (unless the dieter is stuck in a plateau or is extremely metabolically resistant). Many successful Atkins followers report that after they gained experience with the diet, they could stop counting carbohydrate grams because they had become competent at estimating their carbohydrate intake.

Ketosis is another benefit often cited by Atkins diet followers. For the most part, the followers of Dr. Atkins' plan embrace ketosis and view it as a helpful tool for losing weight. The most common reason Atkins followers like ketosis is that it suppresses their appetite and squelches their carbohydrate cravings. Not being hungry is one of the most frequently mentioned benefits of the diet. Many Atkins followers also state that they like how ketosis provides them with visual confirmation that the diet is working (through urine tests). Other reasons Atkins followers like the Atkins plan is that they experience many of the health benefits claimed by Dr. Atkins, such as reduced hypertension. (For a list of other benefits, see Chapter 4 of this book.)

While the Atkins diet is widely viewed as a simple plan, it is not without structure, and many people are drawn to it for this reason. Many people are most comfortable when they are given clear parameters and defined boundaries. The Atkins diet boundaries are both simple and clear: First, restrict carbohydrate to the level of ketosis. And second, if you are no longer in ketosis, cut back.

Many people who consider themselves to be seriously addicted to carbohydrate prefer the Atkins diet because of its strict reduction of carbohydrate. Many of them view Dr. Atkins' diet as comparable to the treatments for other addictions. Restricting the offending substance is the key to success. For some, this preference is based on experience. Many of these folks tried other reduced carbohydrate diet plans and found that the more liberal intake of carbohydrate revived their addictions and set them off on a path of uncontrolled eating. For them, following the philosophy that "even a little is a lot" is the best approach.

Along these same lines, some people prefer the Atkins diet because of its cold turkey approach to breaking carbohydrate addiction. As with other addictions, some people prefer to stop all at once and be done with it quickly, while some prefer a more gradual withdrawal. Those who prefer the cold turkey approach choose the Atkins plan because the 14-day induction period immediately breaks their carbohydrate addiction. Although some of the symptoms associated with this cold turkey withdrawal can be quite uncomfortable, many dieters much prefer to slay that dragon and get it over with, rather than drag it out for a longer period.

In general, the opinion among reduced carbohydrate dieters is that weight loss tends to be faster on Dr. Atkins' plan than on the other plans, and, therefore, people with a great deal to lose seem to be drawn to it. However, the plan is also viewed as causing weight to be lost in stages, with more stalls and plateaus along the way. Despite the plateaus, Atkins followers often say that they remain with the plan because they find it very satisfying and easy to follow.

The Carbohydrate Addict's Diet

The Carbohydrate Addict's Diet, another best-selling low carbohydrate diet book, was published in 1993. Two research scientists, Dr. Rachael F. Heller, who holds a Ph.D. in research psychology, and Dr. Richard F. Heller, who holds a Ph.D. in research biology, wrote the book. The diet sprang from Dr. Rachael Heller's struggles with her weight. She developed the diet, followed it to lose a significant amount of weight, then used it to maintain the loss for more than 14 years. As a testimonial to the effectiveness of her diet, Dr. Heller recounts the story of how she used the principles outlined in the book to lose approximately 150 pounds. The Carbohydrate Addict's Diet grew from her accidental discovery that restricting the amount of carbohydrate in her diet led to weight loss. Her husband, Dr. Richard Heller, who also lost weight on the diet, assisted Rachael in applying the physiological principles that refined the diet to its present state. In 1983, they founded the Carbohydrate Addicts' Center in New York City and began using the diet to treat other overweight people. They claim a phenomenal 80 percent success rate not only in reducing weight, but in maintaining the weight loss among their clients.

The Plan

The Hellers agree with the other reduced carbohydrate diet book authors that the primary cause of obesity is an overproduction of insulin brought on by too much carbohydrate in the diet. The Hellers also support the theory that when we ingest too much carbohydrate, our level of insulin becomes chronically elevated, causing our blood sugar levels to drop too low. They believe that when our blood sugar levels drop too low, hunger results, and a couple of hours after a meal, we are compelled to eat again. Further, they believe that because our insulin level remains chronically elevated, our nervous system does not release serotonin, a brain chemical that lets the body know it is no longer hungry. Because serotonin is not released, or is released in very small amounts, we do not feel satisfied and our hunger quickly returns. A vicious cycle of weight gain develops.

Carbohydrate Addicts

The unique characteristic of the Hellers' diet and what separates it from the other reduced carbohydrate diet plans is the authors' distinctive theory that 75 percent of all people who are overweight are carbohydrate addicts. This belief is the foundation of their plan, as its name implies. They believe that some foods, particularly simple carbohydrates, are addictive substances much the same as alcohol and drugs. According to their theory, carbohydrate addicts are overweight people who have an intense, compelling, recurring, and gripping hunger and craving for foods rich in carbohydrate, primarily foods composed of simple, refined sugar. The Hellers believe that carbohydrate addiction is similar to other addictions in that the intensity of the cravings escalates over time.

The Hellers do not believe that all overweight people are carbohydrate addicts, nor do they believe that their diet works for all overweight people. They include a quiz in their book and on their web site that serves as a guide in determining whether a person is a carbohydrate addict or not. The quiz also indicates the degree of carbohydrate addiction. According to the Hellers, carbohydrate addiction can range from mild to severe, with symptoms escalating along a continuum.

Controlling the Addiction

The Hellers believe there are three primary methods by which carbohydrate addicts can control their addiction, and these methods constitute the major doctrine of their plan. First, carbohydrate addicts must limit the number of times per day they eat carbohydrate. In *The Carbohydrate Addict's Diet*, dieters are instructed to eat only three meals per day. Snacks between meals are strictly forbidden (unless the goal is to maintain weight rather than to lose it). Two of the three meals, known as Complementary Meals, must contain little or no carbohydrate. The Hellers do not provide guidance on the amount of carbohydrate, calories, protein, or fat that can be eaten with the Complementary Meals except to say that these meals should be low in fat and high in fiber, and have portions that are average sized.

Second, carbohydrate intake is allowed only during the third meal, known as the Reward Meal. The Hellers strongly disagree with the other reduced carbohydrate diet book authors, who believe it is best to spread the carbohydrate intake evenly throughout the day. The Hellers believe that eating carbohydrate at all three meals causes a constant release of insulin, which is detrimental to carbohydrate addicts. According to their theory, insulin released throughout the day sets carbohydrate addicts up for failure by perpetuating the destructive, addictive cycle that causes them to crave carbohydrate.

The Hellers also recommend limiting carbohydrate intake to only one meal because they believe that the pancreas releases insulin in two distinct stages. This is important because they believe that the amount of insulin the pancreas releases in the first stage is based on the amount of carbohydrate ingested in *previous* meals. Therefore, by restricting carbohydrate intake in two of the three meals, the first insulin release (at the third meal) is minimized.

The third method by which carbohydrate addicts can control their addiction, according to the Hellers, is by limiting the length of time of the Reward Meal. The Hellers instruct carbohydrate addicts to eat their Reward Meal in 60 minutes or less. Their rationale is that the second release of insulin occurs about 90 minutes after a meal begins. By limiting the Reward Meal to 60 minutes, the amount of insulin released in the second stage is lessened.

The Hellers advise dieters to establish routines in which the Reward Meal is the same meal each day, whether it is breakfast, lunch, or dinner. In their book *The Carbohydrate Addict's Diet,* they broadly state that the quantity and type of carbohydrate eaten in the third meal are not restricted. They state that dieters can eat any carbohydrate-rich food they wish in any quantity they wish. They say only that the Reward Meal should be "balanced." However, in later books and on their web site, the Hellers narrow these instructions somewhat. They state in *The Carbohydrate Addict's LifeSpan* and on their web site that they did not intend for the Reward Meal to be an unbalanced "carbohydrate binge." They meant for it to be a "balanced feast." Their updated recommendation is to begin the Reward Meal with approximately 2 cups of salad followed by a meal composed of one-third protein, one-third low carbohydrate vegetables, and one-third carbohydrate-rich food (including dessert). Dieters do not need to limit the amount of fat they eat during the meal, but the Hellers caution them to choose polyunsaturated oils and olive oil as much as possible. If dieters remain hungry, they can consume an unlimited amount of additional food at the meal. However, they should eat more of all three of the food groups, not just carbohydrate.

Addiction Triggers

The Hellers introduced the now popular concept of addiction triggers in the book. They believe that certain foods, people, events, and situations disrupt carbohydrate addicts' biochemistry and trigger eating episodes (commonly known as binges) that can lead to weight gain. They encourage dieters to identify their own personal triggers, and they offer several strategies for conquering them. In fact, they devote several chapters of the book to the psychological and emotional challenges of weight control.

Fat

The Hellers strongly recommend reducing the amount of all fats and cholesterol in the diet, including in the Reward Meals. They recommend using olive oil, polyunsaturated oils, and spray oil when cooking. They warn against eating saturated fats, tropical oils, and cholesterol (although they loosen these restrictions in later books). In fact, they state their diet is completely compatible with the U. S. government's recommendations for low fat, low cholesterol diets.

Fiber

The Hellers agree that fiber is an important part of the diet. For Complementary Meals, they recommend choosing high fiber vegetables from a list they provide in the book. For Reward Meals, they recommend high fiber foods of the dieter's choice. They do not mention the glycemic index, nor do they discuss the technique of subtracting fiber grams from total grams of carbohydrate (see Chapter 4 of this book).

About the Book

Of all the books written to date about low and moderate carbohydrate dieting, *The Carbohydrate Addict's Diet* is probably the most distinctive in its approach. This enormously popular book broke ground in that it popularized the pioneering concept of carbohydrate addiction. While its basic theory closely matches those of the other reduced carbohydrate books, it is different in two ways. First, the Hellers applied the psychological framework of addiction to explain the tendency to overconsume carbohydrate. Since the introduction of this book, the concept of carbohydrate addiction has become part of mainstream vocabulary in the world of reduced carbohydrate dieting, and many other reduced carbohydrate diet experts have adopted it.

Second, the Hellers recommend eating all carbohydrate in one 60-minute meal, rather than spreading it evenly throughout the day. This concept is unique to the Hellers.

Because of Dr. Rachael Heller's background in counseling and her personal experience in being substantially overweight, there is a strong undercurrent of psychological support in this book. She devotes a substantial amount of time to providing psychological comfort. The basic theme is, "You have failed before, but it is not your fault." In fact, the book is dedicated to, "the untold numbers of carbohydrate addicts who, deep down, have always known it was not their fault."

Rachael and Richard Heller are scientists, and their research background is clearly reflected in this book. It is scientific in its approach, yet it is not overwhelming in its detail. The complexity of this book is beyond that of a primer, but it is not so complex that most readers will get lost in the detail.

The book provides sample meal plans and recipes suitable for the Complementary Meals. It also contains a carbohydrate gram counter and an extensive bibliography.

Why Followers Like the Diet

One of the strongest attractions for most Heller followers is the core philosophy of the diet. Many of them say that when they first heard the term "carbohydrate addict" and read the book, it was as though a key had been handed to them to unlock a lifelong mystery. They felt they were reading about themselves. These people strongly identify with the addiction explanation put forth by the Hellers and, as a result, believe that approaching their weight problem within this framework is the key to success for them.

One of the more pragmatic reasons Heller followers like the plan is that it allows the daily Reward Meal. While the two Complementary Meals make the diet very similar to the Atkins diet and the Protein Power diet because they allow little to no carbohydrate, being able to eat any food they wish at least once per day is extremely inviting for many people. People who are cooking for a family like the fact that the Reward Meal is flexible enough to allow them to prepare one meal, rather than one for them and a second one for their family. Some followers of other plans, such as the Atkins diet and the Protein Power diet, borrow the Reward Meal concept from the Hellers and use it to control "planned cheats," such as when they are at special occasions and parties.

The Carbohydrate Addict's Diet is most attractive to people who prefer a gradual approach to carbohydrate withdrawal, rather than the cold turkey approach. While many Heller followers report that in the early stages of the diet, they thought of little else than what they would eat in their next Reward Meal, they say that over time their addiction waned and they ate less and less carbohydrate. Eventually, they stopped focusing on the Reward Meal, and their overall carbohydrate intake dropped. Many followers say that was when they knew their carbohydrate addiction was broken.

The plan is also attractive to people who want *some* flexibility in their diet plan—but not too much. While the plan is very structured overall, having the flexibility to include any high carbohydrate food in their Reward Meals keeps followers from feeling deprived of their favorite foods. Any time they have a strong craving for a particular food, they know they are no more than 24 hours away from being able to eat it, and this helps keep the craving under control. Many people report that their cravings for that "I-must-have-it-or-die" food weaken after a while on the diet. In essence, the food loses its attraction because it is no longer forbidden.

While the general consensus among the reduced carbohydrate dieters is that weight loss is somewhat slower on the Carbohydrate Addict's Diet, the Hellers claim that plateaus are less frequent and of shorter duration on their diet than on the other reduced carbohydrate diet plans. They credit this relative lack of plateaus to the Reward Meal. They say that the carbohydrate allowed in the Reward Meal prevents the body from going into "starvation mode" and reaching a point of slow weight loss. Carbohydrate Addict's Diet followers who acknowledge that weight loss tends to be slower on this plan than on other low carbohydrate diet plans say that the benefit of having Reward Meals is worth the slower loss.

The Zone

Dr. Barry Sears, a well-known research scientist with a Ph.D. in research biochemistry, published *The Zone* in 1995. He became interested in the prevention and reversal of heart disease because of a family history of serious heart disease and premature death. He began his reduced carbohydrate research in 1984 and wrote *The Zone* in 1995 after he came to the conclusion that cardiac disease, along with obesity, hypertension, atherosclerosis, increased cholesterol, diabetes, depression, alcoholism, chronic fatigue syndrome, premenstrual syndrome, and even cancer, was either caused or negatively influenced by unbalanced, high carbohydrate diets.

The Plan

Dr. Sears describes the Zone diet as adequate in protein, low in fat, moderate in carbohydrate, and low in calories. Like the authors of the other reduced carbohydrate diet books, Dr. Sears believes that too much insulin is produced after eating excessive carbohydrate. He agrees that sustained high insulin levels and suppressed glycogen levels lead to obesity. He believes the only way to control the balance of insulin and glucagon is to achieve a balance of carbohydrate and protein in a low calorie diet.

Eicosanoids

Dr. Sears also believes that a group of powerful hormones known as eicosanoids are just as important as insulin and glucagon in controlling weight. He explains that the eicosanoids are master hormones that control virtually every body function. He believes that diet influences the balance of "good" and "bad" eicosanoids, and too much carbohydrate negatively influences this critical balance. When carbohydrate and protein are properly balanced in the diet, the eicosanoids are properly balanced in the body. Dr. Sears believes that when this beneficial balance occurs, a heightened state of mental and physical functioning is the result. He refers to this state as the Zone, hence the name of the book. "The Zone" is a term that comes from the world of professional sports and athletic competition, but it is applicable to general health, according to Dr. Sears. The foundation of the Zone diet is the premise that food is a powerful tool that places a person in the Zone, even more effectively than drugs. Dr. Sears states that when dieters eat Zone-appropriate, balanced meals, they will be "in the Zone" for approximately six hours. By repetitively eating proper meals, dieters can be perpetually in the Zone.

Portion Control

Dr. Sears believes there are two effective methods to influence the balance of the eicosanoids. The first is to control meal sizes, since he believes excess calories stimulate the production of insulin. He instructs dieters to eat three small meals and two small snacks per day because he strongly believes it is important to spread food intake evenly throughout the day. His theory is that small, frequent meals cause small, frequent releases of insulin. He believes large meals are detrimental in that they cause large insulin releases and upset the insulin-glucagon balance and the "good-bad" eicosanoid balance. He states that each meal should be no more than 500 calories and each snack should be no more than 100 calories. He cautions dieters not to go more than five hours without eating.

Carbohydrate and Protein

The second method that Dr. Sears recommends for influencing the balance of "good" and "bad" eicosanoids is to maintain a beneficial ratio of dietary protein and carbohydrate. He calls this recommendation the foundation of his diet and refers to it as the cardinal rule. The cardinal rule is: Eat 3 grams of protein for every 4 grams of carbohydrate at every meal and snack. This ratio works out to 0.75 gram of protein per 1 gram of carbohydrate.

Dr. Sears allows some flexibility in this ratio. Depending on their biochemistry and activity levels, dieters can eat between 0.6 and 1.0 gram of protein per gram of carbohydrate. Dr. Sears believes that eating small meals that contain the proper protein-to-carbohydrate ratio allows dieters to control not only the balance of insulin and glucagon, but also, and more importantly, the balance of the eicosanoids.

Dr. Sears strongly advocates using the glycemic index to choose carbohydrate sources. He recommends vegetables and fruits that have a low glycemic index to minimize insulin releases.

In addition to warning dieters against consuming too much carbohydrate, Dr. Sears also cautions them not to eat too much protein. He believes that excessive dietary protein causes kidney strain when the protein is broken down to be stored as fat. He also believes that too much protein leads to calcium loss. Most importantly for dieters who want to lose weight, Dr. Sears believes that excess protein inhibits weight loss because protein stimulates insulin release. His concern about eating too much protein is another primary reason he recommends a balance of carbohydrate and protein at every meal and snack.

Fat

Dr. Sears describes his diet as low fat, yet he does not believe that fat should be restricted to very low levels. He believes that fat is the primary and best fuel for muscle. In addition, he believes that an adequate fat intake is important for losing weight. First, when fat is eaten with carbohydrate, it slows the absorption of the carbohydrate into the bloodstream and reduces the amount of insulin that is released. Second, fat improves the taste and satisfaction of the meal. Third, when fat is eaten, the stomach signals the brain that the body is satisfied, and hunger is diminished as a result. Fourth, "good" fats are essential for the production of "good" eicosanoids.

Dr. Sears encourages dieters to eat monounsaturated fats, such as olive oil, canola oil, olives, macadamia nuts, and avocados. He says these fats should make up the bulk of the fat in the diet. He cautions against eating saturated fats, and he strongly warns against taking in arachidonic acid, a compound found in egg yolks, organ meats (including processed deli meats), and fatty red meats. He believes that arachidonic acid leads to the manufacture of "bad" eicosanoids and calls arachidonic acid restriction a central theme of his diet.

Adding fat to the cardinal rule of protein and carbohydrate intake results in the following recommendation: Eat 7 grams of protein per 9 grams of carbohydrate per 1.5 grams of fat. (Athletes, however, need to eat more fat than this.) Dr. Sears states that every meal and snack should have this ratio of protein to carbohydrate to fat. To simplify this rule, he encourages dieters to think of each of these units as a "Zone block." In other words, 7 grams of protein is a protein block, 9 grams of carbohydrate is a carbohydrate block, and 1.5 grams of fat is a fat block. Using this approach, each meal and snack should have a ratio of one protein block to one carbohydrate block to one fat block. He states that if his diet were described in terms of a percentage of calories, his diet would be composed of 40 percent carbohydrate, 30 percent protein, and 30 percent fat.

Total Intake

Dr. Sears recommends that dieters base the amount of carbohydrate and fat in their diet on the amount of protein required by their body. In the book and at his web sites, he provides a detailed method to determine protein need based on lean body mass, body fat percentage, and activity level. He advocates eating as closely as possible to the minimum protein figure that results from this method. He encourages dieters not to eat significantly below or above the recommended protein level. He then instructs dieters to determine the amount of carbohydrate and fat to be added to the diet by calculating the grams of each allowed, using the ratios presented above.

Ketosis

Dr. Sears strongly warns dieters against restricting carbohydrate to the point of inducing ketosis. He believes that carbohydrate is necessary for proper brain function and that ketosis deprives the brain of its primary fuel source. He believes ketosis results from a breakdown of lean body mass (not fat stores) during a period of starvation. He believes that ketone bodies are removed from the body through the urine, breath, and feces because they are abnormal biochemicals that are harmful to the body. He also believes that ketosis causes basic changes in the cells that enable them to regain weight more readily after keto-sis ends.

About the Book

People who want scientific detail on why and how re-duced carbohydrate diets work love *The Zone*. It answers the critics of some of the other reduced carbohydrate diet books who say there is not sufficient scientific data to sup-port the theories behind reduced carbohydrate diets.

The level of detail in this book springs from Dr. Sears' extensive education and experience in research biochem-istry. He states early in the book that one of his goals in writing the book was to provide a comprehensive resource on diet for physicians, nutritionists, and health profession-als. As a result, he has built a strong scientific infrastruc-ture and demonstrates a solid scientific case for the reduction of carbohydrate in the diet. The book contains a wealth of scientific and biological information about how the body is affected by diet, including the benefits of re-ducing carbohydrate intake.

Having said that, the flip side is that the book can be a bit complex, and readers who are not health or nutrition professionals may find it too detailed at times. In response, Dr. Sears has written a companion book, *A Week in the Zone*, which presents the diet in a simpler fashion.

The Zone is a multi-issue book that covers a lot of ground on how reduced carbohydrate diets affect several aspects of health, not just weight loss. People who want to use reduced carbohydrate dieting for reasons other than weight control can find the information they need in this book.

The book also provides several useful tools for Zone di-eters. It contains detailed worksheets that walk dieters through the calculation of lean body mass and minimum protein requirements. A table that guides dieters in defining food blocks is included as well (for example, 1.5 ounces of uncooked chicken breast is one protein block). The book also contains a selection of Zone-favorable menus and recipes, as well as a table that compares the average body fat percentages of selected sports-related professionals. It provides a comparison of the Metropolitan Life tables for ideal weight in 1959 and 1983. It provides a table of groupings of the glycemic index of select foods. It also provides instruction on how to contact the technical support team. Lastly, it contains an extensive bibliography.

Why Followers Like the Diet

Generally, the Zone diet appears to appeal the most to advanced dieters and people with scientific or healthcare training, although people from all walks of life use it successfully. People who are detail-oriented and want a highly structured diet that gives them precise control and a deep understanding of the nutrition they provide their bodies gravitate to it. For example, Dr. Sears' diet is popular among athletes who are very serious about using nutrition to optimize their athletic performance. In fact, Dr. Sears is a nutrition coach for several Olympic athletes. Many people who follow Dr. Sears' diet say the promise of improved athletic performance is one of the main reasons they follow the diet.

Of all the reduced carbohydrate plans, Dr. Sears' diet is the most structured. There not only are guidelines for the amount of carbohydrate, protein, fat, and calories that should be ingested at each meal and each day, but there are also guidelines that govern the relationship of each of these factors to the others. Dr. Sears' followers find the benefits of the diet are worth the effort required to plan meals, plan menus, and calculate the correct ratios of carbohydrate, protein, fat, and calories.

This scientific orientation of the Zone diet is also evident in the official Zone web sites. The discussion boards tend to have a technical and scientific focus. In fact, there are busy official technical support sections at the Zone web sites. These sections allow Zone followers to ask technical questions and get answers from a team of scientists, physicians, and Zone-certified instructors. (Yes, there is a course one can take to become a Zone-certified instructor.) The web sites also provide several tools that Zone followers need, including spreadsheets that calculate Zone blocks, meal profiles, minimum protein recommendations, and body fat percentage calculations.

The Zone diet is attractive to people who believe that high carbohydrate, low fat diets lead to obesity, but do not believe that simply restricting carbohydrate to very low levels is the remedy. Dr. Sears' followers often describe the Zone as moderate and balanced. Generally, the diet is viewed as being more liberal in total carbohydrate intake than the other low carbohydrate plans in that it does not limit carbohydrate intake to very low levels. Zone followers like using the glycemic index to guide them in choosing a variety of low glycemic fruits and vegetables.

Dr. Sears' diet appeals to people who believe that low calorie diets are valuable in supporting overall health. They often cite studies concluding that people who have lower calorie intakes enjoy longer and healthier lives.

Sugar Busters!

Three New Orleans physicians and a Fortune 500 chief executive officer published *Sugar Busters! Cut Sugar to Trim Fat* in 1995. Originally, this book was released as a self-published book. Its popularity was obvious right away: It sold over 300,000 copies largely by word of mouth. Given this impressive early success, it was no surprise when it appeared on *The New York Times* bestseller list in 1998.

The three physicians—Dr. Morrison C. Bethea, a cardiac surgeon, Dr. Samuel S. Andrews, an endocrinologist, and Dr. Luis A. Balart, a gastroenterologist—joined H. Leighton Steward, the chief executive officer of a Fortune 500 company who successfully implemented the diet and maintained his weight loss for five years, to write the book. All three of the physicians actively practice medicine, and they recommend the diet to their patients.

The Plan

The authors present a simple, moderate carbohydrate diet plan in this uncomplicated, straightforward book. Of all the reduced carbohydrate diet plans, with the possible exception of NeanderThin, the Sugar Busters! plan is probably the least structured. The authors state that their philosophy in writing the book was to provide dieters with basic nutritional information that would allow them to make informed food choices, not to dictate their diets to them, and this philosophy is evident throughout the book.

These four authors agree with the authors of the other reduced carbohydrate diet books that the primary cause of obesity, diabetes, insulin resistance, heart disease, and hypertension is excess carbohydrate in the diet. In fact, they refer to refined carbohydrate as toxic. They further agree that the overproduction of insulin that results from too much carbohydrate is the primary mechanism that leads to these major health problems. When it comes to the specifics of weight loss, they believe that not only does an overproduction of insulin create excess body fat, but it leads to obesity because it also suppresses the production of beneficial glucagon and, therefore, actually inhibits the breakdown of body fat. They emphasize that even low levels of insulin prevent the breakdown of body fat. Therefore, they say, the key to losing weight is to control the secretion of insulin by controlling the amount and type of carbohydrate in the diet.

Although the authors of *Sugar Busters!* depart somewhat from traditional medical advice by recommending that dieters limit the amount of carbohydrate in their diets, they do not stray far from conventional medical advice when it comes to other aspects of the plan. They are largely silent on the ranges of carbohydrate, protein, and fat that should be consumed, and they state that it is unnecessary to count sugar grams, fat grams, or protein grams when the diet is followed properly. However, in interviews dated May 25, 1998 (posted on the Sugar Busters! web site), the doctors are quoted as saying the diet should be composed of 40 percent carbohydrate, 30 percent fat (10 percent saturated fat), and 30 percent protein. The recommendations of 30 percent overall fat intake and 10 percent saturated fat intake closely match the current recommendations of the general nutrition and medical communities.

The authors agree that the calorie theory is not valid for weight loss, yet they emphasize that portion control is very important and they provide uncomplicated instructions to limit food intake. The amount of food eaten at each meal should be limited to that which fits in the flat portion of an average (not oversized) plate (not including the flared edges). They caution against eating second helpings. They recommend spreading the intake of carbohydrate evenly throughout the day. They instruct dieters to eat at least three meals, each of which should contain moderate amounts of carbohydrate. They also recommend snacking on low glycemic fruit between meals. They do not support eating carbohydrate during only one or two large meals per day. They believe that spreading the total carbohydrate intake over several meals will cause less insulin to be released than eating an equivalent amount of food in one or two meals. They do not support the practice of skipping meals or going for prolonged periods without eating because they believe this alters the insulin response and makes weight gain more likely to occur.

The authors cite studies they claim support their belief that the calorie theory is not valid for weight loss. In fact, they claim the calorie theory is counterproductive in that it promotes undereating, which eventually slows metabolism. They also believe low calorie diets are self-defeating in that few people can sustain undereating for a long period and find that when they return to eating a normal volume of food, the weight they lost returns.

The authors agree with the other reduced carbohydrate diet book authors that insulin resistance is a major contributor to obesity, type II diabetes, and heart disease because as the body loses its sensitivity to insulin, it must produce more to be effective. They assert that at least 50 percent of insulin resistance can be reversed through their diet.

Carbohydrate

The book does not provide guidance on the amount of carbohydrate that should be eaten other than saying that no one food should contain more than 3 grams of refined sugar per serving. This gives the impression that the plan is much more liberal in carbohydrate intake than some of the other reduced carbohydrate diet plans, although it is not expressly stated.

In keeping with their philosophy of not dictating a diet to their followers, they do not give a limit on the number of grams of carbohydrate that can be eaten per day. Instead, they emphasize the quality and type of carbohydrate that dieters should eat. The authors strongly support the glycemic index (a statement at their web site calls it the foundation of the diet). The authors instruct dieters to avoid foods with simple, refined sugar because they have high glycemic index values and to choose fruits, vegetables, and whole grains with low glycemic index values. The idea is to control blood sugar levels by eating low glycemic index foods rather than by simply restricting all carbohydrate to low levels. In fact, the Sugar Busters! plan is not intended to restrict carbohydrate intake to the point that ketosis occurs, and the authors do not mention ketosis in their book. However, Dr. Bethea stated in an interview (posted on the Sugar Busters! web site) that ketosis should be avoided because, he believes, the kidneys, heart, and muscles do not function well in ketosis.

Protein

The authors believe that balancing the amount of protein eaten each day is crucial to the success of the program. On one hand, they state that eating an adequate amount of protein improves the insulin-glucagon balance in two ways: First, dietary protein does not stimulate insulin release, and second, it does prompt the release of the beneficial hormone glucagon. They recommend eating a minimum amount of protein based on total body weight. The formula they use is 1 gram of protein for each kilogram (2.2 pounds) of body weight. They strongly recommend eating plants, lean meats (including trimmed red meats), fish, fowl, eggs, cheese, and nuts as the primary sources of protein and avoiding fatty meats. They recommend the protein sources be baked, grilled, or broiled rather than fried.

On the other hand, they caution dieters against eating too much protein, as they believe that excess protein is converted to glucose through a process known as glucogenesis and that, therefore, body fat can be increased by eating too much protein.

Fat

The Sugar Busters! plan calls for moderate dietary fat intake, meaning that while the authors do not endorse low fat dieting, they do not allow unlimited fat intake either. Overall, they recommend that 30 percent of total calories be derived from fat and saturated fat limited to 10 percent of all calories. They do not provide guidance on the number of fat grams that should be eaten each day.

They strongly caution that not all fats have the same effect on the body, and they make distinctions between healthy and unhealthy fats. The key, they say, is to take in enough healthy fats to meet the body's needs without overdoing it. In fact, they assert that healthy fats are important for many critical body functions, including hormone production. They also state that a few healthy fats—namely, monounsaturated fats (including olive oil)—actually lower cholesterol levels. The fats they include on their list of healthy fats are monounsaturated fats such as olive oil, some nut oils, and omega-3 polyunsaturated acids (fish oils).

On the other hand, they caution dieters against eating unhealthy fats—namely, saturated fats and some polyunsaturated fats—and they state that they are very concerned about excessive consumption of saturated fat in particular. Although red meat is often high in saturated fat, they say eating some lean, trimmed red meat is acceptable.

Fiber

The authors often repeat their belief that insoluble fiber in the diet has a strong positive impact on weight loss. They believe that insoluble fiber slows the digestion of carbohydrate and prevents large, sudden increases in the blood glucose levels. This, in turn, prevents large, sudden insulin releases. In fact, insoluble fiber is the main reason they believe so strongly in the glycemic index. A high fiber content usually causes foods to have a low glycemic index value.

Exercise

Exercise is an important part of the Sugar Busters! plan, according to the authors. They emphasize that exercise should be moderate and regular, and they caution against strenuous exercise. They believe that overexercising backfires because the body will use glucogenesis to convert protein to glucose to raise the blood sugar levels to provide energy to the muscles that are under stress.

About the Book

The authors of this brief, simple book state that their philosophy is to provide readers with basic information that will allow them to make informed food choices. This mission is clear throughout the book; it is written in a down-to-earth, uncomplicated style that clearly explains the benefits of reduced carbohydrate dieting without going into a great deal of detail. The authors include some information on the impact of carbohydrate and insulin on heart disease, diabetes, and other illnesses, but for the most part, the book is focused on using the diet to lose weight.

The book provides a listing of foods that are and are not acceptable on the Sugar Busters! plan, including suggestions for substitutions for the foods that are not acceptable. It provides 14 days of sample meal plans and a chapter of recipes. It also contains a glossary of nutritional and medical terms and a bibliography.

Why Followers Like the Diet

Sugar Busters! followers often say they like the plan because it is a moderate, middle-of-the-road plan. They often cite their belief that the diet is safe and healthy as one of the primary reasons they chose the diet. One of the reasons Sugar Busters! followers have a high degree of comfort with the safety of the plan is that the recommendations do not depart dramatically from the medical advice that is familiar to them. Except for the restriction of carbohydrate to low glycemic foods, the advice (such as on the amount and types of protein and fat that should be in the diet) is closely in line with the current government recommendations. Because the plan is not viewed as a dramatic departure from current medical advice, it is not often criticized in the popular media, as are some of the lower carbohydrate diet plans.

Sugar Busters! followers also like the plan's unstructured nature. Dieters who are comfortable with a great deal of flexibility and freedom in making food choices are attracted to this plan. The followers of this diet say the plan has the added benefit of allowing them to easily plan meals and menus that also work for their family; they do not need to prepare separate meals for themselves and others. Many dieters who lost weight on the lower carbohydrate plans use the Sugar Busters! diet for weight maintenance because of its flexible nature.

For the most part, Sugar Busters! followers obtain the structure they need by using the glycemic index to make their carbohydrate food choices. Most of them agree that the glycemic index is an easy tool for choosing foods to eat. They also say that shopping is easy and that the plan is less expensive than the diet plans that advocate very low levels of carbohydrate. By including some sources of carbohydrate, the overall cost of the groceries is lowered. (Many dieters state that low carbohydrate diets can be expensive because the sources of protein and fat that are recommended tend to be costly.) And finally, dieters who are not in a big hurry to lose weight are also drawn to this plan because the weight loss is generally slower. Their philosophy is that they are less likely to regain the weight this way.

Dr. Bernstein's Diabetes Solution

Dr. Richard K. Bernstein published *Dr. Bernstein's Diabetes Solution: A Complete Guide to Achieving Normal Blood Sugars* in 1997 and added a much-needed dimension to low carbohydrate dieting. In his book, Dr. Bernstein tells the story of how he discovered that low carbohydrate dieting could control his diabetes over 20 years ago. However, because he was an engineer and not a physician at the time of his discovery, he was not able to capture the attention of the medical or nutritional community to explain his approach. Therefore, at the age of 41, he enrolled in medical school, and he has devoted his subsequent medical career to the treatment of diabetes. A summary of Dr. Bernstein's book is included here because diabetics who practice low carbohydrate dieting frequently cite Dr. Bernstein as a valuable resource for them.

Dr. Bernstein strongly believes that the presence of a "thrifty gene" causes some individuals to be predisposed to excessive fat production and weight gain. He believes it is Mother Nature's mechanism to protect us from periods of famine. However, during times of prolonged feast, he believes this thrifty gene leads not only to the development of obesity, but to type II diabetes as well. He also strongly supports the theory that some individuals are addicted to carbohydrate in much the same way that some people are addicted to drugs.

The Plan for Weight Loss

While the focus of this book is on instructing diabetics how to use low carbohydrate dieting to control their blood sugar levels rather than to lose weight, Dr. Bernstein includes a chapter that assists diabetics in creating a diet for weight loss. Dr. Bernstein recommends weight loss for all diabetics because he believes that losing body fat improves the control of type II diabetes by reducing insulin resistance. For those diabetics who are dependent upon insulin injections to control their blood sugar levels, he believes that losing body fat significantly reduces the need for additional insulin injections.

Dr. Bernstein recommends eliminating all simple carbohydrate and restricting complex or long-acting carbohydrate to a point that allows control of the blood sugar levels. The degree of restriction required is highly individualized; some diabetics will require mild to moderate restriction, while others will require severe restriction. Dr. Bernstein states that once diabetics have determined the degree of carbohydrate restriction that is necessary for them to control their blood glucose levels, they should begin to reduce their level of protein intake to lose weight (if they are not losing weight already). He instructs diabetics to reduce their protein intake at one meal per day by one-third for a week. If they do not begin to lose at least one pound per week, they should reduce their protein intake by one-third at a second meal. They should continue this protein reduction process until a point is reached where weight loss occurs at a rate of approximately one pound per week. However, Dr. Bernstein cautions diabetics not to restrict their level of protein intake to less than five grams per day, as restricting protein below this level will lead to serious malnutrition.

Dr. Bernstein refers to low fat diets as the "big fat lie" and strongly states that he does not believe obesity is related to excess dietary fat intake or that dietary fat affects blood sugar levels. Therefore, he does not restrict fat intake in his diet plan.

Exercise

Dr. Bernstein strongly recommends lifting weights to build lean body mass and muscle. He believes not only that muscle burns more calories than does fat, but that adding muscle increases the body's sensitivity to insulin and therefore reduces insulin resistance. He also states that natural endorphins are released during weight lifting that reduce appetite.

About the Book

The book has a wealth of information about diabetes, including its origins and the history of its treatment. The author clearly explains how low carbohydrate dieting can control blood sugar levels and reverse some of the damage already inflicted by the disease. It is a comprehensive book, yet it is written in a simple, easy-to-read style. If you are a diabetic who wants to lose weight and gain better control of your blood glucose levels, this book is a must-read; it is packed with great information on how the effects of diabetes can be brought under control and weight loss can be achieved through low carbohydrate dieting.

Why Followers Like the Diet

Reduced carbohydrate dieters who are currently diabetic or are at high risk for developing diabetes later love *Dr. Bernstein's Diabetes Solution* because it specifically addresses their needs. While the authors of the other reduced carbohydrate diet books often provide a discussion of how their diet improves the management of blood sugar levels for diabetics, it is often highly summarized. *Dr. Bernstein's Diabetes Solution* provides the detail that many diabetics need, particularly those who are on oral hypoglycemic medications or insulin injections. Bernstein followers often state that they have a high degree of trust in the efficacy and safety of his diet because he is a physician who struggled with severe (type I) diabetes for the whole of his life.

Protein Power

Two practicing physicians, Dr. Michael R. Eades and Dr. Mary Dan Eades, published *Protein Power* in 1995. *Protein Power* became a best-selling book and has remained on *The New York Times* best-seller list for over six years.

The Eades are physicians who practice exclusively in the specialties of bariatric medicine (weight loss) and nutritional medicine. They founded and continue to practice at the Colorado Center for Metabolic Medicine in Boulder. They emphasize the benefits not only of restricting carbohydrate intake, but also of eating adequate amounts of protein, hence the name of the book. Because of the influence of this popular diet plan, some nutritionists and the popular media began to refer to reduced carbohydrate diets as high protein diets rather than low carbohydrate diets.

The Plan

Although the Eades' program is often compared to Dr. Atkins' diet, it also incorporates many of the theories presented by Dr. Sears in *The Zone*. They, like most of the authors who write on the subject, support the theory that obesity and many other serious illnesses are primarily caused by an overconsumption of carbohydrate leading to high insulin levels. They further believe that low blood glucose levels cause the pancreas to release glucagon, which in turn causes body fat to break down. Like Dr. Atkins, they believe that restriction of carbohydrate to a low level is necessary to correct the problem. They advocate ketosis as a method by which fat breakdown can be quickly accomplished, although they do not require it. While they say that ketosis can occur when carbohydrate intake is restricted to the degree they recommend, they counsel dieters not to be concerned if it does or does not happen. They prefer dieters to be on the cusp of ketosis. Like Dr. Sears, they emphasize the impact of the diet on the eicosanoid balance in the body, but they do not believe that restricting carbohydrate intake to low levels causes an imbalance in them.

The Eades describe their plan as a carbohydrate restricted, moderate fat, and adequate protein diet. The goal of the Protein Power diet is to maximize glucagon production while minimizing insulin production, and the Eades believe that controlling the diet is the only way in which this goal can be accomplished. They believe the key strategy is adequate protein intake, restricted carbohydrate intake, and moderate fat intake.

Three Phases

The Eades recommend three dieting phases. The first two phases, called the intervention phases, are recommended for weight loss. In Phase I Intervention, carbohydrate is restricted to 30 grams or less per day. This phase is recommended for people who have more than 20 percent of their body weight to lose or have one of the other serious illnesses caused by excess insulin production.

Phase II Intervention is recommended once dieters have less than 20 percent of their body weight to lose or after their serious illness has significantly improved. Dieters can skip Phase I and begin the diet at this stage if they have less than 20 percent of their total body weight to lose or their goal is generalized health improvement. At this stage, carbohydrate intake is restricted to 55 grams or less per day.

Once dieters have achieved their weight loss goal, they can enter the maintenance phase of the diet. This phase is recommended when dieters are within 5 percent of their goal weight. The authors recommend a slow transition to the maintenance phase because a sudden increase in carbohydrate is likely to disturb the insulin-glucagon balance established during Phases I and II. They recommend that carbohydrate intake be raised by 10 grams or less every five to seven days. Carbohydrate intake should be raised until it is roughly equivalent to the minimum daily protein requirement or the point is reached where weight loss stops. For dieters who are physically active, carbohydrate intake may be increased by up to one-third more than protein intake. If weight gain occurs during maintenance, dieters should return to Phase I dieting until the extra weight is lost. These dieters can then progress to Phase II eating for a week before returning to maintenance level eating.

In all three phases, the Eades recommend that carbohydrate intake be spread evenly throughout the day to avoid sudden insulin releases. For example, in Phase I, each meal should contain 7 to 10 grams of carbohydrate, for a total of 21 to 30 grams of carbohydrate per day. The Eades assert that saving all carbohydrate for one meal is detrimental because it causes sudden increases in insulin production.

Protein

In all three phases, the Eades instruct dieters to consume at least their minimum recommended amount of protein each day. The book provides a detailed method to arrive at this figure. The figure is based upon lean body mass and level of activity. The Eades do not give guidance regarding the maximum amount of protein to be eaten each day. Instead, they instruct dieters to eat more protein if hungry, but not to eat until overfilled.

Fat

The Eades do not believe that dietary fat intake should be reduced to the levels currently recommended by the medical community. They do not recommend restricting fat intake or counting fat grams, but they do make a distinction between healthy and unhealthy fats. They recommend that the bulk of dieters' fat intake come from fats such as olive oil, nut oils, fish oils, avocados, and butter. They instruct dieters to avoid fried foods, hydrogenated fats, trans fats such as margarine, and arachidonic acid (if a dieter is sensitive to it).

Fiber

The Eades do not support the glycemic index as a method for choosing carbohydrate sources. In fact, they devote a portion of their book to pointing out the flaws in the glycemic index approach, and they discourage dieters from using it. Instead, they recommend a simpler approach of subtracting the grams of fiber from the total grams of carbohydrate in food. They use the term "effective carbohydrate content" to identify the difference between these two counts. The idea is that fiber is not digestible and, therefore, need not be counted in the daily carbohydrate count. They recommend taking in at least 25 grams of fiber per day from food sources. This is to encourage dieters to obtain their carbohydrate from sources such as vegetables, rather than from refined sources.

Nutritional Supplements and Exercise

The Eades devote an entire chapter of their book to the importance of nutritional supplements in improving overall health and promoting weight loss. Another chapter is devoted to exercise. They strongly advocate exercise as part of their program and emphasize the benefits of resistance training (weight lifting).

About the Book

Protein Power builds a bridge between the simplicity of *Dr. Atkins' New Diet Revolution* and the complexity of *The Zone*. It is clearly more detailed in its explanation of low carbohydrate diets than Dr. Atkins' book, but not nearly to the degree of Dr. Sears' book. It is a good middle-of-the-road book that presents a full explanation of the science of low carbohydrate dieting in a way that is understandable by those who are not health professionals.

While the authors focus on weight loss in this book, they do spend a considerable amount of time discussing the benefits of low carbohydrate dieting on general health and many chronic diseases. They have written a second book, *The Protein Power LifePlan*, in which the topics of chronic illnesses such as heart disease are more fully discussed.

Protein Power also provides several useful tools, including detailed worksheets that walk dieters through the calculation of lean body mass and minimum protein requirements. It provides a brief restaurant dining guide, a week of sample menu plans, a chapter of recipes, and an extensive bibliography.

Why Followers Like the Diet

For the most part, the Protein Power diet is viewed as very similar to the Atkins diet, probably because both diets recommend a carbohydrate intake in the range of 30 to 60 grams per day and advocate ketosis as a method for weight loss. Many low carbohydrate dieters refer to the two diets interchangeably, and the followers of these two plans easily intermingle in Internet discussion groups.

Therefore, all the reasons people like the Atkins diet apply to the Eades diet. With the combination of adequate protein intake, high fiber vegetable intake, and ketosis, most Protein Power followers say they are very satisfied with the food they eat and do not feel hungry. Serious carbohydrate addicts who want to approach their diet through a "cold turkey" withdrawal and consistent reduction in carbohydrate also like the plan.

With that said, there are some important differences between Protein Power and the Atkins diet. Many people who choose to follow Protein Power view the diet as a little more liberal than the Atkins diet because ketosis is not required (although it is not discouraged either). Many dieters say they considered the Eades' emphasis on eating fiber and low carbohydrate vegetables in their decision. They like the method of deriving the effective carbohydrate content by subtracting the fiber count from the total carbohydrate count. They also view the Eades' recommendation of getting at least 25 grams of fiber each day as an attractive aspect of the diet.

Weight loss is widely viewed as being faster on the Protein Power plan than on the other reduced carbohydrate diet plans. However, stalls and plateaus tend to affect Protein Power followers, and there is always a steady stream of discussion among the followers on how to break them.

The Schwarzbein Principle

Dr. Diana Schwarzbein, a practicing physician from Santa Barbara, California, published *The Schwarzbein Principle: The Truth About Losing Weight, Being Healthy, and Feeling Younger* in 1999. Prior to writing this book, Dr. Schwarzbein was best known for her work as the founder of the Endocrinology Institute of Santa Barbara and her association with actress Suzanne Somers. (She advocates

Ms. Somers' *Somersizing* weight loss plan.) Dr. Schwarzbein specializes in metabolic problems, diabetes, osteoporosis, menopause, and thyroid dysfunctions.

Dr. Schwarzbein brings a holistic perspective to reduced carbohydrate dieting in that she covers the impact of high carbohydrate diets on aging, depression, eating disorders, and several degenerative diseases, in addition to obesity. In fact, although she states that weight loss is not the ultimate goal of her program (the primary focus is achieving optimum health), she frequently repeats her assertion that her program produces less body fat and more lean body mass. (After all, losing weight is the first benefit she mentions in the book's subtitle.)

She agrees with the other reduced carbohydrate diet book authors that excess body fat is a direct result of too much carbohydrate in the diet. She also agrees that low calorie diets and low fat diets are not valid methods for either losing weight or achieving health. She agrees that excess carbohydrate consumption causes the body to overproduce insulin. Other factors she names as a cause of elevated insulin levels are stress, chronic dieting (especially yo-yo dieting and low fat dieting), skipping meals, caffeine, alcohol, aspartame, saccharin, tobacco, steroids, stimulants (such as ephedrine), lack of exercise, excessive or unnecessary thyroid hormone replacement, and many over-the-counter and prescription drugs.

Although Dr. Schwarzbein agrees with many of the theories promoted by the other low carbohydrate diet book authors, she resists the low carbohydrate label that is sometimes used to describe her diet plan. She much prefers to describe her plan as a balanced, moderate carbohydrate diet. In fact, she strongly cautions dieters against very low carbohydrate diets. She believes that the low insulin levels that occur when carbohydrate is restricted to very low levels are detrimental to health. For example, she believes that low insulin levels lead to depression because one of the functions of insulin is to prompt serotonin releases in the brain. She says that when insulin is not present, serotonin is not released and depression results. She also believes that low insulin levels lead to fatigue, insomnia, and loss of bone mass.

Another reason she cautions dieters against very low carbohydrate diets is that she strongly believes ketosis is harmful because ketone bodies lead to imbalanced hormone systems.

Dr. Schwarzbein repeatedly emphasizes that the goal of any weight loss program should not be simply to lose weight, but rather to achieve a beneficial body composition by reducing body fat and building lean body mass. She is critical of low calorie, low fat, high carbohydrate diets because she says that the increased insulin levels that accompany them promote an unhealthy ratio of body fat to lean body mass. Because fat and protein are restricted on low fat diets, lean body mass is lost. Because increased carbohydrate intake prompts insulin releases, body fat is often maintained and the lean body mass–to–body fat ratio shifts unfavorably. This unfavorable ratio backfires in that it lowers the metabolic rate, which in turn causes a predisposition to gain weight. Dr. Schwarzbein feels strongly that it is not possible to lose more than 2 pounds per week without losing lean body mass and damaging the body's metabolic rate. Therefore, she recommends losing weight at a rate of 1 to 2 pounds per week.

Dr. Schwarzbein strongly believes that the medical community has incorrectly concluded that many chronic illnesses are genetic when in fact they are caused by excessive carbohydrate intake and insulin production. She speaks a great deal about achieving balances in health and in life to prevent and cure several degenerative diseases, and she advocates a natural diet made up of whole, unprocessed foods to do so. She believes that highly processed foods and artificial food products damage cells and lead to illness. In fact, she says that one of her goals in writing this book was to convince readers to stop eating artificial and chemical-laden foods.

The Plan

Dr. Schwarzbein presents her plan in two stages: the healing program and the maintenance program. The goals of the healing program are to achieve a proper balance between body fat and lean body mass, improve or reverse insulin resistance, reverse accelerated metabolic aging, and improve or reverse chronic illnesses. The goals of the maintenance program are to maintain the improvements that were achieved in the healing program, prevent recurrence or development of illnesses, and optimize health.

In both phases, Dr. Schwarzbein believes dieters should strive to keep insulin and glucagon in balance, rather than simply attempt to keep insulin levels low. She states that insulin is released after eating carbohydrate, glucagon is released after eating protein, and neither insulin nor glucagon is released after eating fats and nonstarchy vegetables. (She defines nonstarchy vegetables as those vegetables that contain less than 5 grams of carbohydrate per half-cup serving.) Therefore, she advocates eating the following four basic food groups at every meal: nonstarchy vegetables, complex carbohydrate, protein, and good fats. She believes that eating these four food groups together at every meal balances insulin and glucagon releases. She calls this approach the Schwarzbein Square. She believes strongly that the Schwarzbein Square approach is much preferable to the U.S. Department of Agriculture (USDA) food pyramid. In fact, she strongly criticizes the USDA food pyramid because she believes it minimizes the fats and proteins that are critical for building important body tissues while encouraging the overconsumption of carbohydrate.

Dr. Schwarzbein instructs dieters to eat according to the Schwarzbein Square rather than the USDA food pyramid to achieve a proper balance of insulin and glucagon. She emphasizes the necessity of eating carbohydrate and protein together at every meal because she strongly believes that the optimal insulin-glucagon balance is disrupted by an unbalanced intake of carbohydrate and protein. For example, if carbohydrate is eaten alone or in excess, too much insulin is released and the insulin-glucagon balance is disrupted. On the other hand, if protein is eaten alone or in excess, the insulin-glucagon balance is disturbed by too much glucagon. Nonstarchy vegetables and healthy fats are neutral in that they do not cause either glucagon or insulin releases, so do not disrupt the insulin-glucagon balance. Therefore, a substantial amount of both should be eaten at every meal.

Dr. Schwarzbein also states that it is important to combine these four food groups at every meal because protein, fat, and fiber slow the digestion of the carbohydrate, thereby lessening the risk of excessive insulin releases. She frequently cautions dieters that eating carbohydrate without the other three groups leads to overeating because the body has no natural mechanism that limits the amount of carbohydrate that is eaten at one time. Therefore, it is very easy to overeat carbohydrate when it is eaten alone.

Carbohydrate

Dr. Schwarzbein recommends different amounts of carbohydrate in the healing program and in the maintenance program. In fact, the amount of carbohydrate is the only difference between the two phases. In the healing program, she recommends eating carbohydrate at a level that is slightly below the dieter's current metabolic needs to promote the loss of body fat. Once the proper body fat composition has been achieved, Dr. Schwarzbein recommends eating slightly higher levels of carbohydrate in the maintenance program.

Dr. Schwarzbein does not recommend the same amount of carbohydrate intake for all dieters. Instead, she presents ranges of carbohydrate intake for different body compositions, body weights, and activity levels. For example, she provides guidelines for underweight, normal weight, slightly overweight, and overweight people. She further breaks down each of these categories by degree of physical activity: sedentary, somewhat active, active, and extremely active. She instructs overweight dieters to eat between 15 and 30 grams of carbohydrate per meal, depending upon their activity level. Dieters who choose to eat at the lower end of the carbohydrate range per meal (15 grams) should also eat two snacks of 7.5 to 15 grams of carbohydrate per snack. If depression becomes a problem, she instructs dieters to increase their carbohydrate intake by an additional 7.5 grams per meal.

Dr. Schwarzbein instructs dieters to choose their sources of carbohydrate carefully. She warns dieters that carbohydrate should be derived only from natural, unprocessed sources, rather than refined, man-made sources, such as processed food products. She defines natural carbohydrate sources as whole grains, legumes, fresh vegetables, and unprocessed fruits. She refers to these as "real foods" because they can be eaten in their natural state or after being cooked by simple, common methods. She provides several extensive lists of acceptable and unacceptable foods in the book. When it comes to choosing carbohydrate sources that are not on her lists, she advocates using the glycemic index because the carbohydrate sources that she recommends have naturally low glycemic index values.

As part of the Schwarzbein Square approach to eating, Dr. Schwarzbein says that every meal should include plenty of fresh nonstarchy vegetables. Because nonstarchy vegetables have low glycemic index values, high nutrient contents, and a lot of fiber, she says their carbohydrate content does not need to be counted in the daily carbohydrate counts.

Generally, Dr. Schwarzbein discourages dieters from weighing and measuring foods because, she says, the practice causes an unhealthy psychological fixation on food. However, she concedes that it is necessary to weigh, measure, and count carbohydrate at the beginning of the diet. Her reason is that the body does not have a natural mechanism for limiting the intake of carbohydrate, as it does for protein and fat. Therefore, it is very easy to overeat carbohydrate. By weighing and measuring food at the beginning, dieters learn how to mentally estimate the amount of carbohydrate they can consume.

Protein

Dr. Schwarzbein does not limit the amount of protein that can be eaten in either phase of her program. She believes it is not necessary to limit protein intake since the body naturally limits the amount of protein that can be eaten at one time. She instructs dieters to count protein grams only if they are concerned they are not eating enough of it. Generally, she recommends an average woman ingest at least 60 to 70 grams of protein per day and an average man at least 70 to 80 grams of protein per day. She instructs dieters to eat protein at every meal.

Fat

Dr. Schwarzbein spends a significant portion of her book outlining her arguments against low fat diets. She strongly believes that good fats are essential for health and fitness because fat contributes to the healthy development of cell membranes, hormones, and other vital tissues. She often states, "The more good, healthy, natural fats people eat, the healthier they become." She believes a lack of good fats actually contributes to illnesses, insulin resistance, and accelerated aging. Therefore, Dr. Schwarzbein believes it is unnecessary and unhealthy to restrict fat intake.

Dr. Schwarzbein instructs dieters to eat good fat at every meal and to eat as much of it as they feel their body needs. She differentiates between the various fat sources by dividing them into two groups: good fats and bad fats. As the labels imply, she believes that some fats are healthy and some are not. She instructs dieters to avoid bad fats. She includes on her list of bad fats any fats that have been modified by man (she calls them "damaged fats"), such as trans fats, oxidized fats, and hydrogenated fats. She also includes polyunsaturated fats and other fats that have been damaged through heating, such as in deep-frying. She states the following oils are damaged unless they are pure-pressed or cold-pressed: corn, cottonseed, poppyseed, safflower, sesame, soybean, sunflower, and walnut.

Dr. Schwarzbein includes as good fats those natural

polyunsaturated fats that have not been processed or heated. Other good fats are saturated fats (yes, saturated fats) and monounsaturated fats. Virtually all fats in their natural forms, such as olive oil, flaxseed oil, butter, mayonnaise, eggs, and avocados, are included on her good fat list. She cautions that even good fats can be damaged by heating and, therefore, should not be heated to extremes. She states that all cooking should be done at low, even temperatures. She warns dieters never to eat deep-fried foods.

Dr. Schwarzbein does not limit the amount of fat in her diet. She states that it is not necessary to do this because fat does not stimulate insulin releases and the body limits the amount of fat that can be eaten at one time.

Serotonin

Dr. Schwarzbein includes a great deal of information in her book about the effects of diet on the levels of serotonin in the brain. Serotonin is a natural brain chemical that is critical in such brain functions as maintaining an elevated mood. Normal and high levels of serotonin are associated with elevated moods and high energy levels, while low levels are associated with depression and low energy levels. Dr. Schwarzbein agrees with the theory that sugar is a stimulant and is addictive, and she associates its addictiveness with the release of serotonin. She says sugar functions much the same as other stimulants do in that, at first, a person gets a "rush" of serotonin after eating sugar, but over time, the amount of serotonin released with each sugar ingestion becomes less and less. Dieters are compelled to eat more and more sugar to get the same effect as they experienced in the beginning. The net effect of eating sugar (and taking other stimulants) is that serotonin becomes depleted and the brain chemistry becomes imbalanced.

Dr. Schwarzbein believes that the Schwarzbein Square approach supports the optimal production of serotonin. By eating adequate amounts of fat and protein, dieters give their bodies enough of the building blocks needed to produce serotonin. She also believes that complex, natural carbohydrate produces an appropriate amount of insulin for serotonin production. She believes that without insulin, serotonin becomes depleted, and depression and fatigue follow.

Exercise

Dr. Schwarzbein believes that exercise is a vital component of any healthy lifestyle. Specifically, she believes that exercise reverses insulin resistance. She recommends mild to moderate exercise and cautions against exercising as a justification for overeating carbohydrate. She points out that exercise may burn off excess carbohydrate, but it cannot burn off the excess insulin that accompanies it.

Vegetarians

Dr. Schwarzbein includes a chapter on reduced carbohydrate dieting for vegetarians. She has also published a cookbook for vegetarians.

About the Book

Dr. Schwarzbein brings the perspective of a naturalist to the reduced carbohydrate world. While her primary premise is that high carbohydrate diets contribute to obesity and other serious illnesses, she also spends a significant amount of time recommending a natural, additive-free, unprocessed diet.

While weight loss is an important theme in her book, it

is not the sole focus of it. Dr. Schwarzbein spends a great deal of time discussing the benefits of reduced carbohydrate diets on chronic and degenerative illnesses, and on aging and depression. The wide range of subjects makes this book a great resource for people seeking a solid understanding of the benefits of moderate carbohydrate dieting beyond weight loss. She also includes information on the effects of the diet on children and adolescents, making it a valuable resource for the parents of children with weight issues.

While Dr. Schwarzbein covers a significant amount of science and biology in the book, she worked with a professional science writer, Nancy Deville, to ensure that the book would be readable and understandable. As a result, it is simple and easy to read, yet provides a comprehensive explanation of her moderate carbohydrate diet.

The book includes a chapter for vegetarian dieters. It also contains four weeks of sample menu plans and a chapter of recipes.

Why Followers Like the Diet

Since the book is a relatively recent release, a consensus on the full benefits of the *Schwarzbein Principle* has not yet fully developed. To date, the most common reason people cite for following the plan is that it is a good tool to maintain the weight they have already lost. Generally, the book gets good reviews among reduced carbohydrate dieters, especially among people who want to more fully understand the overall health benefits of reduced carbohydrate diets.

NeanderThin

In 1999, Ray Audette published his book *NeanderThin: Eat Like a Caveman to Achieve a Lean, Strong, Healthy Body* and spawned a "naturalist" movement among reduced carbohydrate dieters. Also known as the Paleolithic Diet, Hunter-Gatherer Diet, Stone and Spear Diet, and Caveman Diet, Mr. Audette's plan provides a whole new perspective for modern man. ("Paleolithic" is the term used by scientists to describe the age when man relied upon hunting and gathering for food. It was a time before agricultural techniques were developed.)

The NeanderThin diet was born out of Mr. Audette's struggle with two chronic and devastating illnesses— rheumatoid arthritis and diabetes. He developed his diet plan after becoming frustrated with the medical care he was receiving for these illnesses. Mr. Audette, who is a member of Mensa, responded by researching the causes of autoimmune disorders and diabetes, and the effects of diet upon them. He came to the conclusion that our modern diet of high carbohydrate, highly processed food is the cause of most of the chronic and degenerative diseases of our day. He concluded that our bodies are best suited for a natural, pre-agricultural, non-technology-dependent diet. He chose to mimic the diet of Paleolithic man and was astounded at the immediate, positive results. His arthritis symptoms dramatically decreased, his blood sugar levels came under control, and he lost 25 pounds.

The Plan

Mr. Audette's plan is simple and straightforward: Eliminate from the diet any food that does not occur in nature. Mr. Audette instructs dieters to eat only those foods that can be hunted or gathered from nature and digested in their raw state. With the exception of meat, if a food requires any sort of technology to transform it from inedible to edible, it should not be eaten. In other words, if dieters cannot hunt or gather the food, it should not be part of their diet.

Mr. Audette does not present his diet in the traditional model of recommending a range of intake for carbohydrate, protein, and fat. Instead, he simply applies the no-technology rule and allows any foods that pass the test. He describes the diet as a loose set of guidelines rather than a rigid plan. Although he does not limit the amount of carbohydrate in the diet, his plan is naturally low in carbohydrate because there are only a few sources of simple sugar in nature. He summarizes the NeanderThin plan in what he terms "The Ten Commandments" of the diet: five groups of foods that should not be eaten (forbidden foods) and five groups of foods that should be eaten (permitted foods).

Forbidden Foods

In general, Mr. Audette restricts any food that requires technology to be edible. He specifically lists the following five groups of forbidden foods and gives the rationale for why each should be avoided.

- *Grains*. Mr. Audette recommends that all grains, including wheat, rice, oats, barley, rye, and corn, be eliminated from the diet for several reasons. First, he cites studies which conclude that when grains are ingested, health deteriorates. Second, he feels that grains do not pass his natural rule because they are not edible without significant milling and processing.

Third, he argues that grains are unhealthy. Not only are wheat and corn the most common allergens in our diet, but corn often contains potent cancer-causing fungi known as aflatoxins.

- *Beans*. Mr. Audette warns against eating all forms of legumes because they contain natural ingredients known as alkaloids that act as pesticides in nature and have deleterious effects on humans.

- *Potatoes*. Potatoes also contain harmful alkaloids and should be excluded from the diet, according to Mr. Audette.

- *Dairy*. Mr. Audette views dairy products, especially milk, as being highly processed and feels they should be avoided, since it is only technology that makes them edible and safe. He also points out that milk is the third most common allergen, after wheat and corn.

- *Sugar*. Other than honey, Paleolithic man rarely ate simple sugar, according to Mr. Audette. While Mr. Audette does not forbid eating fruits, he cautions dieters that the fruits of today have been affected by technology through selective breeding for sweeter taste and larger size. The fruits of Paleolithic man were smaller and less sweet than the fruits of today.

In addition to these five groups of forbidden foods, Mr. Audette also recommends eliminating alcohol from the diet because of its potentially damaging effects on the liver, stomach, and kidneys. He also places coffee on his list of forbidden foods, since it cannot be consumed in its natural state.

Mr. Audette recommends complete abstinence from,

not just restriction of, these five groups of forbidden foods. He states that these foods are addictive (especially the carbohydrate they contain), and eating just a little will cause strong cravings for them later. He uses as an analogy the fact that abstinence is the only effective method of treating alcohol addiction.

Permitted Foods

In addition to listing forbidden foods, Mr. Audette lists five groups of foods that should be eaten.

- *Meat and fish.* Mr. Audette strongly encourages dieters to eat meat, including red meat, poultry, fish, crustaceans, and small mammals such as rabbits and squirrels. He believes eating meat is essential to health and this food group should not be excluded from the diet. He cautions dieters to avoid processed meats that contain additives and preservatives. He states that eating meat is not only essential but natural, since all primates are carnivores.

- *Fruits.* While Mr. Audette encourages dieters who are striving to optimize their health to eat fruits, he also cautions dieters who are attempting to lose weight to limit the amount and types of fruits they eat. He recommends that these latter dieters reduce or eliminate some fruits such as peaches, plums, apples, pears, and oranges because they have a higher carbohydrate count than other fruits such as tomatoes and melons. He feels that fruits are best eaten fresh and raw. He instructs all dieters to avoid canned and preserved fruits, including jellies and jams.

- *Vegetables.* Mr. Audette recommends that vegetables make up a significant portion of the diet. As with fruits, he recommends that vegetables be eaten in their raw, uncooked state because of their superior content of vitamins and nutrients. However, he says that cooked vegetables are only slightly less nutritious and can be included. He cautions dieters to remember that some foods commonly thought of as vegetables, such as corn and yams, are not allowed.

- *Nuts and seeds.* Mr. Audette encourages the consumption of nuts and seeds because he believes they are important sources of fat and calories. He defines nuts as the "seed of a tree" and warns that peanuts are not allowed, since they do not meet this definition. He also does not include cashews in the list because cashews must undergo significant processing before they are edible.

- *Berries.* Mr. Audette advocates eating berries in their natural raw form. He states that they are a good low carbohydrate food for people who want to lose weight.

Fat

In addition to the five permitted food groups, Mr. Audette actively encourages dieters to eat an adequate amount of fat. He does not support the current medical recommendations that fat should be restricted and states that fat should be the primary source of calories in the diet. He believes fat is essential for critical body functions, as a source of energy, as a stabilizer of blood glucose levels, and for providing satisfaction from meals. He warns that attempting to limit fat intake on the NeanderThin plan is a mistake because fatigue and hunger will result.

Mr. Audette encourages dieters to include sources of the essential fatty acids as much as possible. He recommends that the sources of dietary fat be olive oil, avocados, lean meat, seafood, and nuts. He cautions dieters to avoid hydrogenated oils and oils derived from any forbidden foods, such as corn oil and soybean oil.

About the Book

The book presents a well-written case for the Paleolithic diet. Mr. Audette clearly walks the reader through the history of the development of man and explains how and why our diet has a major impact on our health. He presents easy-to-understand information about our digestive system as compared to those of other species, including the lower primates. He clearly explains why he believes eating highly processed foods damages our bodies, using a comparison to modern-day hunter-gatherer tribes in Africa as evidence.

The book is not focused solely on weight loss. In fact, weight control is not its central theme, despite its title. However, Mr. Audette does spend a significant amount of time discussing the Paleolithic diet as a weight loss method.

The book contains a foreword by Dr. Michael Eades, coauthor of *Protein Power.* Dr. Eades clearly supports the principles of the diet, although he points out that it is more restrictive than the diet he and his wife recommend in their book *Protein Power.*

The book offers a five-week program that includes exercise suggestions, menu plans, and recipes. It also contains a bibliography.

Why Followers Like the Diet

The book is a relatively new release, and a full following of supporters has not yet developed. However, the plan gets good reviews overall among reduced carbohydrate dieters. Naturalists are drawn to this diet for its "Mother Nature supplies all we need" message. NeanderThin followers most often cite improved health as the primary reason they try to stick with the plan. Many persons who have difficulty controlling their blood sugar levels practice the plan. Although the plan is widely believed to be more restrictive than the other low and moderate carbohydrate plans, NeanderThin followers say that the improved health that results makes it worthwhile.

Thin for Good

The latest contribution to the world of reduced carbohydrate diet books comes from Dr. Fred Pescatore, who published *Thin for Good: The One Low-Carb Diet That Will Finally Work for You* in 2000. Dr. Pescatore, who was the associate medical director of the Atkins Center for Complementary Medicine for five years, founded and is now serving as the medical director of the Centers for Integrative and Complementary Medicine in New York and Dallas.

The Plan

In *Thin for Good*, Dr. Pescatore adds several dimensions to the reduced carbohydrate diet. First, he provides not only a reduced carbohydrate eating plan, but a psychological support plan as well. He states that he developed the psychological dimension of the diet out of his personal experience as an overweight person and his professional experience as a physician treating obesity. He identifies 11 emotions he believes affect dieters' eating patterns: anger, frustration, sadness, fear, understanding, trepidation, envy, boredom, relief, joy, and contentment.

Dr. Pescatore spends a significant amount of time discussing and recommending a technique he calls mind-body medicines. This technique involves daily meditations designed to give dieters the psychological tools they need to develop healthy attitudes toward food and body weight. He provides 30 days of these daily meditations to get dieters started.

Second, he addresses the differences in dieting between the genders, a topic not covered in the other reduced carbohydrate diet books. His premise is that women and men react to dieting differently, both physically and emotionally, and his plan addresses those differences.

Third, he addresses the different stages of life in his plan. He defines four stages for women: beginners, young women, perimenopausal/menopausal women, and postmenopausal women. He defines three stages for men: beginners, weekend warriors, and the experienced. Therefore, he does not present one plan for all dieters. Instead, he presents several plans designed for the different genders and stages of life. He provides quizzes for both women and men to help them determine their stage of life and adapt his diet plan to their own needs.

Dr. Pescatore has two overall phases in his diet plan. First, for all dieters, he recommends an initiation phase lasting at least 30 days, perhaps more if there is a large amount of weight to be lost. The second phase, the forever phase, is intended for lifetime maintenance of the weight loss. In both of these phases, the amount of carbohydrate, protein, and fat that is recommended depends on gender and stage of life.

Dr. Pescatore advocates portion control, which he believes is an important factor in losing weight and maintaining weight loss.

Carbohydrate

Dr. Pescatore states that there are differences among the types of carbohydrate, just as there are differences among the types of fats. He states that some sources of carbohydrate are good and some are bad. He recommends only complex, high fiber carbohydrate sources, such as low carbohydrate vegetables, whole grains, brown rice, whole grain pasta, some nuts, seeds, and some legumes. He recommends using the glycemic index as a tool for selecting carbohydrate sources.

Protein

Dr. Pescatore describes protein as the cornerstone of his diet. He recommends that protein intake be balanced with carbohydrate and fat intake to achieve insulin balance. He provides guidance on how much protein to ingest in each of the seven plans. While he recommends that the source of protein be red meat, game animals, fish, poultry, cheese, and eggs, he places some restrictions within each category.

Fat

Like his counterparts, Dr. Pescatore does not recommend that fat be restricted. He does differentiate between good and bad fats, however, and recommends that some fats be used without restriction and some be avoided "at all costs." He also states that some fats are damaged in cooking and, while they are fine in their natural, cold state, they should be avoided when heated. He divides dietary fat into three groups. The first group consists of oils that can be used without restriction, such as olive oil. He calls this group the "gold medal" fats. The second group is made up of oils that should be used sparingly, and he calls these the "bronze medal" fats. The last group, the "lead medal" group, consists of the fats that should be avoided. Included are hydrogenated oils and oils that are damaged when heated. He also recommends that the fat be trimmed from meat because the toxins and antibiotics consumed by animals are stored in the fat.

Putting It Together

Dr. Pescatore presents seven diet outlines for the initiation phase: one outline for each of the four female stages and one outline for each of the three male stages. Within each of these seven outlines, food is divided into six major groups and 13 subgroups:

1. Protein—Red meats, processed meats, fish, poultry, eggs, cheese.
2. Complex carbohydrate—Vegetables, grains, nuts and seeds, legumes.
3. Beverages—Soft drinks, alcohol, milk.
4. Desserts.
5. Condiments.
6. Fruits.

Most of these groups and subgroups are further divided into foods that are allowed and foods that are not allowed. For the foods that are allowed, the portion size is included. Dieters are instructed to choose foods from among the allowed foods in each of the groups, subgroups, and categories to build a dieter-specific diet.

Vegetarians

Dr. Pescatore includes a chapter on reduced carbohydrate dieting for vegetarians.

Nutritional Supplements and Exercise

Dr. Pescatore devotes an entire chapter of his book to the importance of nutritional supplements in improving overall health and promoting weight loss. He devotes another chapter to the important topic of exercise.

About the Book

This book is easy to read and understand, yet it is a comprehensive source of information. For the most part, *Thin for Good* concentrates on the topic of weight loss. In addition, Dr. Pescatore briefly covers the other benefits of reduced carbohydrate dieting.

Thin for Good adds several new dimensions to the traditional reduced carbohydrate diet. The first is that no diet will be successful unless the psychology of dieting is understood. This concept is a strong theme in the book, and every chapter has the psychology of dieting tightly woven into it. Dr. Pescatore's goal with this psychological advice is to provide dieters with detailed instructions for achieving a state of mind that he refers to as "Mind over Calories."

Two other major themes of the book are the differences between men and women in both physiology and psychology when it comes to dieting and the influence of age on dieting. Every chapter takes these differences into consideration.

The book contains 30 days of daily meditations, sample meal plans, and menu suggestions. It also contains 130 recipes.

Why Followers Like the Diet

The book is a new release and has not yet collected a group of supporters.

As you should be able to conclude on your own at this point, although all of the reduced carbohydrate diet book authors begin with the same basic set of theories and assumptions, the way in which they interpret them and use them to correct the underlying causes of obesity are quite different. In spite of these differences, and in many cases because of them, many reduced carbohydrate dieters have developed their own blended approach in which they borrow concepts and ideas from each of the authors and combine them to fashion their own distinctive approach. In fact, much of the discussion on the reduced carbohydrate diet Internet discussion boards relates to just this blending of ideas. In the following chapters, the ideas, concepts, and techniques that have proven successful for the seasoned reduced carbohydrate dieters are presented. I hope you enjoy learning from these seasoned dieters as much as I have.

Table 1.1. Summary Table of Reduced Carbohydrate Diet Plans

	Atkins	Hellers	Sears	Steward et al.	Eades	Schwarzbein	Audette	Pescatore
General Comment	Most popular reduced carbohydrate diet	Introduced concept of carbohydrate addiction; strong psychological support theme	Science-based diet; popular among professional athletes	Simple, unstructured plan that does not stray too far from conventional medical advice	Emphasize the importance of protein; similar to Atkins	Holistic, naturalist diet; strong theme of natural foods and balanced body function	Naturalist diet; introduced concept of Paleolithic-caveman diet	Diet based on gender and life stage of the dieter; strong psychological support theme
Carbohydrate	20 grams in induction phase; restricts in other phases to ketosis	Little in Complementary Meals; liberal in Reward Meals; no guidance on number of grams	4 grams per every 3 grams of protein	No guidance on number of grams; recommend 40% of calories	30 grams in Phase I; 55 grams in Phase II	15 to 30 grams per meal; 7.5 to 15 grams per snack; add more if active or depressed	No guidance on number of grams; restrict to natural sources; omit fruit if goal is weight loss	No guidance on number of grams; provides list of acceptable foods and quantities
Carbohydrate Intake Timing	Spread intake throughout the day	Eat only at daily Reward Meal	Spread intake evenly throughout the day; three meals and two snacks	Spread intake throughout the day	Spread intake evenly throughout the day	Spread intake throughout the day	Does not address	Spread intake throughout the day
Ketosis	Strongly advocates	Do not mention	Strongly discourages	Discourage	Strongly advocate but do not require	Strongly discourages	Does not mention	Does not mention

Table 1.1. Summary Table of Reduced Carbohydrate Diet Plans (Cont.)

	Atkins	Hellers	Sears	Steward et al.	Eades	Schwarzbein	Audette	Pescatore
Protein	No guidance on number of grams	No guidance on number of grams	Foundation of the diet; number of grams based upon body weight, activity level, and body fat percentage	No guidance on number of grams; recommend 30% of calories	Important part of the diet; number of grams based upon body weight and activity level	60–70 grams for average woman; 70–80 grams for average man; believes body has self-limiting mechanism to control protein intake	No guidance on number of grams	Number of grams based upon gender and stage of life
Fat	Unrestricted; warns against making Atkins diet low fat	Recommends low fat intake; states U.S. government recommendations are compatible with CAD	Recommends low fat intake; 1.5 grams of fat per 4 grams of carbohydrate and 3 grams of protein; differentiates between bad fat and good fat	Recommends moderate fat intake; no guidance on number of grams; differentiates between bad fats and good fats	Recommends moderate fat intake; no guidance on number of grams; differentiates between bad fats and good fats	Unrestricted intake of healthy fats; no guidance on number of grams; believes body has self-limiting mechanism to control fat intake	Unrestricted; fat should be primary source of calories in the diet; differentiates between bad fats and good fats	Recommends moderate fat intake; no guidance on number of grams; differentiates between bad fats and good fats
Calories	Unrestricted unless metabolically re-	Unrestricted unless slow loss or stuck	Recommends low calorie in-	Recommends meals that will fit	Unrestricted unless weight loss	Unrestricted; believes body	Unrestricted	Strongly advocates por-

Table 1.1. Summary Table of Reduced Carbohydrate Diet Plans (Cont.)

	Atkins	Hellers	Sears	Steward et al.	Eades	Schwarzbein	Audette	Pescatore
Calories	sistant or stuck in a plateau	in a plateau	take; 500 calories or less per meal; 100 calories or less per snack	in base of plate; no second helpings; no guidance on number of calories	stalls	has self-limiting mechanisms to control protein and fat intake; only restricting carbohydrate is necessary		tion control and recommends serving sizes of allowed foods
Fiber and the Glycemic Index (GI)	Supporting subtracting fiber grams from total carbohydrate count; does not mention GI	Recommends high fiber vegetables; do not mention GI or subtracting fiber grams from total carbohydrate grams	Recommends use of GI and selection of low GI foods	GI is the foundation of the diet; recommends low GI foods	Recommends subtracting fiber grams from total carbohydrate count	Recommends use of GI and selection of low GI foods	Recommends fresh, natural foods; does not mention GI or taking fiber grams from total count of carbohydrate	Recommends use of GI and selection of low GI foods

2
Know What to Expect

Regardless of which of the popular reduced carbohy-drate diet plans you choose to follow, the odds are you will encounter at least one frustrating period of slow loss or a plateau along the way. The goal of this chapter is to give you an idea of what to expect as you progress in losing weight. Some people reach their goals without a hitch, but they are among the lucky few. The very fact that you are reading this book is evidence that you are probably not a member of this fortunate minority. Instead, you are proba-bly like most of us, who are losing weight but are occasion-ally frustrated with our rate of weight loss. Or you may be among those of us who are chronically slow losers and must constantly remind ourselves of the old parable of the tortoise and the hare. This chapter will explain that much of the time there is no reason to be frustrated, as slow weight loss (according to the scale) is not always a sign that you are not losing fat and that your ability to tell the differ-ence will be one of the greatest keys to your success.

All of us, whether or not we are skeptical of the reduced carbohydrate diet when we begin it, have high hopes that it will end our years of trying to lose weight. And we have plenty of reason for elevated expectations. The reduced carbohydrate diet book authors promise a diet that is easier and more effective than any diet we have undertaken in the past. This sounds like heaven in our tired, low fat world. And the promise that our weight loss will happen quickly is even more attractive to us. After reading one (or more) of these popular books, we find our minds and spirits firmly dedicated to this new eating lifestyle. We are eager for our bodies to deliver on the promise the experts make and to deliver on it fast!

The reality is that while the overall satisfaction with the reduced carbohydrate diets is very high, many dieters feel that diet experts may have inadvertently misrepresented the speed at which most of us can expect to lose weight. In fact, in a few of the books, stalled weight loss and plateaus are not even mentioned, giving us the erroneous impression that it will be smooth sailing if only we follow the guidelines faithfully. Of the books that do address slow weight loss and plateaus, the subjects are briefly covered, highly summarized, and buried among several hundred pages of detailed technical information. Many of us simply overlook the discussions.

What to Expect

As a result of reading the great success stories in the popular diet books, our hopes can be quite high when we start. Sadly, many of us quickly learn that the examples given in the books may not represent the speed with which we all can expect to lose weight. One of the reasons is that many of the examples are of persons who had a substantial amount of weight to lose. These dieters usually demonstrate fairly quick and dramatic losses that are very inspiring, but that do not represent the rate of loss that most of us can expect. For example, after Sarah read a low carbohydrate diet book, she was convinced that the diet was a viable option for her to lose the extra 30 pounds she had carried since the birth of her child. She was particularly eager to lose the weight before her 20-year high school reunion. Using the examples in the book as her guide, she quickly calculated that she could lose the 30 pounds in time if she lost 3.8 pounds per week for eight weeks. While she would not have considered this to be possible before reading her chosen book, she now believed it was a reasonable goal. She enthusiastically graphed her plan on her computer as a tool to measure her progress.

By the time Sarah's reunion arrived, she had two months of experience with the diet. Overall, she loved it. She found it satisfying, enjoyable, and easy to maintain. She particularly loved eating many of the foods and recipes of her youth, rather than the low fat fare she had endured for much of her adult life. She was especially happy that she lost weight for her class reunion—but she did not lose 3.8 pounds per week as she had planned. At first, she was very frustrated with her "slow" rate of loss, but she soon learned that her loss was normal and that her expectation had been unrealistic. After she gained an understanding that the average reduced carbohydrate dieter loses around 1 to 2 pounds per week, she was much more satisfied with the progress she had been making.

To ensure that you have realistic expectations, you should consider the amount of weight you wish to lose as compared to your starting weight. This context is particularly important if you do not have much weight to lose because your weight loss is likely to be slower and you are more likely to experience stalls along the way. For a proper perspective, the number of pounds you can realistically expect to lose in any given time period should be estimated as a percentage of your total body weight.

For example, let's say that a married couple begins a low carbohydrate diet on the same day and follows it with the same degree of commitment for six weeks. The husband, who weighs 300 pounds, loses 15 pounds, or 5 percent of his body weight, very quickly and easily. But the wife, who weighs 150 pounds, loses only 7.5 pounds during the same period of time. If only the pounds they lose are considered, it appears the wife is losing weight much more slowly than her husband. In fact, however, both of them lost 5 percent of their total body weight. Therefore, if the wife expects to lose approximately the same number of pounds as her larger husband in the same six weeks, she is likely to be frustrated with the loss she actually experiences. By looking at her loss as a percentage of total body weight, she can celebrate!

This perspective also partially explains why many people find their rate of loss appears to slow as they approach their goal weight. The lighter they are, the fewer pounds they will lose in the same period. For example, a woman begins a diet at 200 pounds. For several months, she loses approximately 2 pounds per week. However, as she becomes lighter and her weight falls to 150 pounds, she finds that she is losing about 1.5 pounds per week. She becomes frustrated. However, her "slowing" weight loss can be explained by looking at it as a percentage of total body weight. By calculating her loss as a percentage of her starting body weight, we see that her weight loss has been constant at 1 percent of her body weight per week. She is incorrectly concluding that her rate of loss has slowed because she is losing 0.5 pound less per week. By looking at her loss in relation to her total body weight, she can enjoy a great feeling of success.

Common Patterns of Weight Loss

While all of us lose weight in our own distinctive, individualized way, there are several patterns of weight loss that you may recognize as your weight loss progresses. If you are fortunate, you will experience only the positive patterns that contribute to easy weight loss, but more likely than not, you will experience a mixed bag of positive and negative patterns that will, over time, smooth out to show real success. This section will give you an overview of what to expect, so as you begin to experience these patterns, you will recognize them for what they are: a normal part of losing weight.

Stalls and Plateaus

No discussion of common weight loss patterns can be complete without first discussing the arch nemeses of all dieters: stalls and plateaus. Stalls and plateaus are dreaded periods of no weight loss that happen even when you do not change your diet or exercise regime. You find that the weight loss tactics that worked well for you in the past suddenly seem to stop working. It seems your body is stubbornly refusing to cooperate, and no amount of pushing or prodding will move it along. There are many theories on why stalls and plateaus occur, but, in fact, no one seems to know for sure. We just know they exist. They happen to all of us, and we hate them.

If weight loss slows dramatically or stops for a short period, the period is referred to as a stall. If the stall becomes prolonged, it is known as a plateau. A plateau gets its name from the visual effect it has on a graph line. It is similar to the outline of a mountainside. As you can see in the graph in Figure 2.1, a typical weight loss graph line resembles

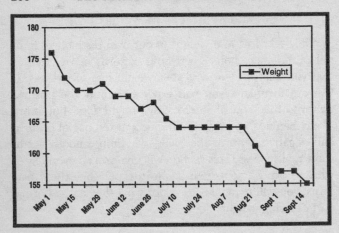

Figure 2.1. A weight loss graph line including a six-week plateau.

the downward slope of a mountain as the weight loss progresses. When the weight stabilizes, the graph line flattens and resembles a plateau. In this sample graph, the line became flattened at 164 pounds for six weeks, thereby producing a temporary flat line, or plateau, before returning to a downward slope.

While most of us are quick to label a period of slow weight loss or a brief stall as a plateau, we are not really in a plateau unless no weight loss occurs for four weeks or more. Therefore, to meet the strict definition of a plateau, weight loss cannot be evident in scale weight, inches, or body fat percentages for a full four weeks. However, for those of us who are in the midst of struggling to lose weight, especially if we have a great deal to lose, any period of no weight loss feels like an eternity. Therefore, many people will refer to themselves as being "plateaued" or "stuck in a plateau" even though their weight loss has stalled for only a short time, sometimes as little as a few days. These are the times when patience truly is a virtue.

The Whoosh Fairy and the Carbo Witch

Stalls and plateaus are so common in reduced carbohydrate dieting that seasoned reduced carbohydrate dieters have developed some fun expressions that reflect their understanding that weight loss often happens in stages. For example, there are joyful times when weight loss is rapid and fat seems to magically melt away. It is not unusual to awaken in the morning and find a sudden, large loss of weight. This blessed event has become affectionately known as a "whoosh." The cause of a whoosh is most often unexplained. As a result, these pleasant events are commonly attributed to a visit from a beloved mythical creature known as the Whoosh Fairy.

For example, Dennis describes the glory of a day the Whoosh Fairy came to visit him. He says that he awoke one morning feeling noticeably lighter. When he stepped on the scale, he found that 2 pounds had disappeared overnight! To make the day even better, he discovered that the whoosh lowered his weight to under the 200-pound barrier. For the first time in years, his weight began with the number 1. The rest of the day, he had an extra spring in his step. His newly washed jeans zipped and buttoned easily. The birds sang marvelously outside his window. The dog was exceptionally well behaved during their daily walk. Even the last remnants of snow melted from the ground in his honor. He had a great day.

On the other hand, there are dark times when weight loss can be agonizingly slow and difficult. These stubborn periods can be extraordinarily frustrating and are attributed to the Whoosh Fairy's evil counterpart, the Carbo Witch. (Others have more colorful names for her, but in the interest of politeness, I will not elaborate!) A visit from the Carbo Witch causes much distress among reduced carbohydrate dieters. This stress is evident in the large amount of discussion among us about how to rid ourselves of the Carbo Witch. Like a visit from an unwelcome relative, visits from the Carbo Witch seem to go on and on, and we become discouraged. These aggravating Carbo Witch stopovers are probably the most common reason people give up and abandon their diet.

The First Whoosh and Stall

Many, though not all, reduced carbohydrate dieters are rewarded immediately with a splendid whoosh in the first two weeks of the diet. This initial loss can be quite large and may amount to as much as 5 percent of our total body weight. Part of this early weight loss is water and glycogen, although not all of it is. In fact, it is so common for the first whoosh to occur right away that many athletes, especially boxers, will use a low carbohydrate diet as a method to quickly lower their weight immediately before a weigh-in. While this first whoosh is a cause of much jubilation for those of us who are lucky enough to experience it, this early success can cause some of us to have inflated expectations that our weight loss will continue at this glorious rate until our target weight is reached. Instead, most of us find that reality arrives soon enough with the first stall, which usually occurs in the third or fourth week of the diet. This stall is so common that it has become something of a rite of passage known as the three-week stall, and seasoned low carbohydrate dieters often caution new dieters to expect it.

For example, Katarina experienced a lot of frustration with her rate of loss in the early stages of her diet. During the first three weeks, she lost 8 pounds, but then she said the diet became a struggle for her. She became frustrated because it seemed the diet had suddenly stopped working. She received great advice from fellow dieters that helped her understand that not only was her pattern of weight loss typical, it was actually to be expected. She learned that it was common for the body to pause in its weight loss for a couple of weeks after the initial loss, and she was reassured that her weight loss would resume if she remained true to the diet. After Katarina divided the 8 pounds she lost by the three weeks she had been on the diet, she realized that she had an average weight loss of 2.7 pounds per week. Katarina began to understand (with the help of her new friends) that she was not failing; she was doing very well.

Front-Loaded Stalls

Another pattern noticed by seasoned reduced carbohydrate dieters is one in which a wonderful whoosh is followed by an aggravating period of slow weight loss. One creative seasoned low carbohydrate dieter coined the phrase "front-loaded stall" to describe this pattern. While some people refer to this period of slow loss as a stall, others argue that it should not be considered a stall at all. Instead, they argue, it should be viewed simply as a period in which our bodies are adjusting to the previous loss. They often encourage stalled dieters to average their weight loss over the entire period to get a more accurate picture of their results. For example, a man experiences a loss of 4 pounds in one week, followed by a week in which he has no loss. Rather than looking at the second week as a stall, he should view the weight loss as being front-loaded, or given to him all at once up front. By looking at the loss as an average over the two weeks, we see that his average weight loss is 2 pounds per week—a rate of loss that should be celebrated.

How Much to Expect

For the most part, average reduced carbohydrate dieters can expect to lose no more than 1 to 2 pounds per week, or about 0.5 to 1 percent of their total body weight per week. Expecting more than this rate of loss sets us up for frustration when none is warranted. Jeremy is a great example of someone who had unrealistic expectations at the beginning of his diet. Jeremy was convinced that his weight loss was too slow because of the prescription medication he was taking. He was frustrated that he was losing "only" 1 to 2 pounds per week when he was planning to lose 4 to 5 pounds per week. He requested information from his low carbohydrate dieting peers about an alternative medication that would break his stall, but the response he received was quite different. Instead, Jeremy learned that he should adjust his weight loss expectations rather than his medication. He learned that while some low carbohydrate dieters will occasionally experience a loss of 4 to 5 pounds in one week, it is unrealistic to expect such a high rate of loss over the long term. He learned that the collective experience of reduced carbohydrate dieters is that 1 to 2 pounds per week was a rate of loss that should be expected and welcomed.

Losing Some Battles, But Winning the War

Not only should we expect a loss of about 1 to 2 pounds per week, we should also view our weight loss over time, not simply by the day or even by the week. The concept of an average weight loss over a period of time is an important one because periods of slow loss and plateaus are certain to occur and should be factored into our expectations. It is human nature for us to overlook the whooshes, since they are usually short, and to dwell on the stalls, which seem to go on forever. By taking a longer view and averaging our loss over a longer period, we get a clearer picture of our success. While our weight may fluctuate up and down with whooshes and stalls in the short term, we often see a downward trend emerge when we view our progress in the longer term. This varied weight loss pattern is demonstrated in Figure 2.2.

The graph in Figure 2.2 demonstrates the great success one man had in reducing his weight from a high of 192 pounds down to 157 pounds in 20 weeks on a popular low carbohydrate diet. As you can see, during the first week on

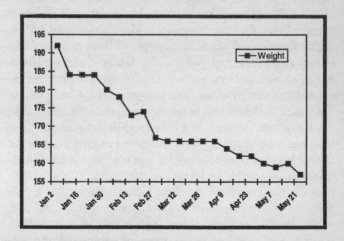

Figure 2.2. The downward trend of weight loss over the long term.

the diet, the man had a wonderful whoosh and lost 8 pounds, but he quickly followed it with a brief stall during which his weight stabilized at 184 pounds for three weeks. Later, he went through several weeks in which he either stayed at the same weight or gained some weight before his weight loss resumed. This is particularly evident in a five-week period during March and April in which his weight stabilized at 166 pounds. Overall, this dieter's average weight loss for the 20-week period was 1.67 pounds per week—a rate that should be expected. Just imagine, had he become frustrated and given up during his long plateau in March and April, he would not have gone on to lose the next 9 pounds and he might even have regained significant weight. Many of us have graphs similar to this one that show there are days or weeks in which it appears we are losing the battle when, in fact, we are winning the war.

For example, Mara found that graphing and averaging her weight over a long period of time dramatically changed her view of her success. Mara was on a reduced carbohydrate diet for 23 months when she began to become discouraged about the length of time it was taking her to reach her goal weight. Her fellow dieters advised her to change her perspective and review her progress by calculating and graphing her average weekly weights for the past 23 months (as is recommended in the book *The Carbohydrate Addict's Diet*). Mara took their advice. She took her weight records and calculated an average weight for each week. For example, if she weighed herself four times in one week and weighed 201, 203, 203, and 202 pounds, she averaged the four weights to arrive at one number that represented her average weight during that week. In this example, her average weight was 202.25 pounds. She repeated this process for each week she was on the diet. Then she plotted the weekly averages on a graph. She was startled by the results. Even in the weeks that she thought her weight loss had stalled, her average weight consistently dropped. Although some of the average weight figures dropped only slightly, they consistently showed a downward trend. Seeing the graph line steadily drop was inspiring for her, and it renewed her commitment to her diet.

You Will Get to Know Your Body

We must also consider that while all of us have the same basic human anatomy and physiology, we are individuals with our own unique reactions and responses. Reduced carbohydrate dieting is no different from any other human process in which there is variability. A good analogy is the growth and development of children. While the milestones and behaviors that can be expected of children at different ages and stages are well defined, no two children move through the same stages in exactly the same way. As most schoolteachers can tell you, the children in their classrooms may be the same age and in the same developmental stage, but they have individual reactions and responses that make them unique. Successful teachers have learned that their relationships with their students must be flexible to account for the differences among the children.

It is much the same with reduced carbohydrate dieting. While the general patterns of how we lose weight and how quickly we lose it can be generally predicted, no two of us will experience the same stage in quite the same way. At first, we learn a great deal about how reduced carbohydrate dieting affects most people, but over time, what we really learn is how reduced carbohydrate dieting affects us. The longer we try, the more we learn and the more we lose.

For example, many dieters say they notice they lose weight "from the top down," meaning their weight loss shows first in their face and neck, then bust or chest, waist, hips, and legs. This is particularly evident to those who regularly track their measurements. Another example is that some people report that once they reach a new low on the scale, their weight stabilizes or fluctuates slightly around that new low figure for a while before they move lower. These folks have learned that they need only to be patient and their weight loss will resume after their bodies adjust to their new low weight.

Other people say their scale gets stuck when they arrive at a weight that they previously maintained for a long time. For example, one woman for years "naturally" weighed 135 pounds. However, after the birth of her first child, she consistently weighed 156 pounds. Following the birth of her second child, she steadily weighed about 178 pounds for a long time before her weight began to slowly creep higher. After she began her low carbohydrate diet, she found she lost weight relatively easily until she reached 178 pounds—the weight she consistently maintained after the birth of her second child. At this point, she was stuck in a plateau for several weeks, but she was patient and she overcame it. Her next plateau was at around 156 pounds— the weight she consistently maintained after the birth of her first child. Once again, she persisted and she broke through the plateau and resumed losing weight. However, once she reached 135 pounds, her previous "natural weight," she found that she could not comfortably go any lower.

Others say that they have become aware of a fun pattern in which their bodies give them a preliminary sign that a whoosh is about to happen. Theo says that on several occasions, he noticed that he needed to tighten his watchband just prior to a whoosh. Marsha says that she always notices that her bra seems looser. Rena reports a kind of "empty feeling" that she is unable to easily explain to us, but it always gives her a "heads up" that her weight loss is about to accelerate. Walter says that he commonly has an uncomfortable, bloated feeling that makes him aware that "a chunk is about to come off."

Your Natural Weight

Some dieters find that as they approach the range of weight that is appropriate for their height, their weight loss slows or plateaus for a long time, perhaps forever. This concept is commonly known as "reaching a natural weight." Our natural weight is the weight at which our body weight stabilizes and refuses to go any lower despite our best efforts. It drives many of us crazy because our bodies seem to have goals that are separate from our own. Our body seems to be happy to have reached its *natural* weight, but we have a goal of reaching our *idealized* weight. If we are very lucky, these two goals are the same, but, most often, they are not. Many people have noticed that their bodies settle at a weight they maintained for a long time in years past. The woman in the example above found that she could not reduce her weight below the 135 pounds she weighed for a long time in years past. For her, 135 pounds was her natural weight. She, however, had her heart set on an idealized weight that was 15 pounds less.

Pamela is a great example of how someone's body may not agree with her goal. She began reduced carbohydrate dieting hoping to lose 39 pounds. In the first three months, she lost 32 pounds, much to her delight. However, as she came within 7 pounds of her goal weight, her rate of loss changed dramatically. Over the next four months, she experienced what she described as a plateau, and she described herself as "the all-time stall record holder." After trying increased exercise and a supplement, she found that she lost a little more weight, but she could not reach her goal weight. Her fellow dieters counseled her that since she weighed only 137 pounds, her body might be telling her that her goal of 130 pounds was not possible. Since 137 pounds was well within the normal range for her height, 137 pounds was most likely her natural weight.

Voice of Low Carb Experience

Most seasoned low carbohydrate dieters find the promise that reduced carbohydrate diets are easy to follow and easy to maintain is fulfilled, especially in comparison to low fat diets. The assurances given by the reduced carbohydrate diet leaders that the diets are more satisfying is supported by actual experience, and overall satisfaction with the diets is high. However, reduced carbohydrate dieters seem to consistently have unrealistic expectations when it comes to how quickly and easily we can expect to reach our goals. We are challenged to understand that it is likely to be an uneven journey for many of us. We are impatient.

So, the best advice from seasoned reduced carbohydrate dieters is this: Adjust your perspective and expect that your weight loss will happen in stages and phases. While you may dream of weight loss that looks like a mature eagle gliding effortlessly on smooth wind currents in a clear blue sky, in reality your weight loss will probably be more like a wobbly new chick struggling to get out of the nest. Know that we all struggle at times, and losing weight slowly drives even the most loyal among us to near madness. For most of us, weight loss comes in fits and jerks with plenty of glitches that keep things interesting.

In addition, while you have every reason to expect great success in losing weight on a reduced carbohydrate plan, it will probably be success that is best measured over time. Expect big whooshes, small losses, stalls, plateaus, and maybe even a few gains as you make your way. And most of all, remember that the single biggest difference between those who are successful and those who are not is that successful dieters are patient, persistent, *and do not give up*. Over time, your body will reveal its own unique responses to reduced carbohydrate dieting, and you will be able to use that information to your advantage.

And last, but not least, do not expect to lose a significant amount of weight quickly if you have a relatively small amount to lose. The lighter your body is, the fewer pounds per week you will lose. If you find that you are not able to drop below a weight that is very close to an appropriate weight range for you, especially if it is a weight that you maintained for a long time in the past, you may have reached your natural weight. If you try to force your weight lower, you may become very frustrated without producing significant results.

Muscle Growth Masks Fat Loss

One of the major advantages of the reduced carbohydrate diets is that they are protein-sparing diets, meaning that nearly all of the weight lost comes from body fat stores rather than from protein-based tissues such as muscle. This advantage is often credited to the fact that protein is a staple in most reduced carbohydrate diets; when we take in adequate amounts of protein, our bodies have the materials they need to build lean body mass.

In contrast, loss of muscle can be a consequence of other diets, especially low fat and low calorie diets, because protein intake is often restricted along with the fat and calories. Many of us spent a long time, even years, on low fat diets. In our efforts to reduce our fat intake to very low levels, we may have inadvertently placed ourselves on low protein diets as well. This is particularly likely if we restricted the amount of meat we ate to cut our dietary fat intake. For some of us, the consequence of prolonged restricted protein intake was reduction in muscle and other lean body mass. Our bodies were simply not able to produce and maintain sufficient muscle because there was not enough protein in our diets to sustain it.

What this means is that if you were previously on a low fat, low calorie diet and you are now eating more protein, you may gain muscle simply because you have returned adequate amounts of protein to your diet. The new protein is stimulating your body to replace the muscle and other protein-dependent tissues that you once lost. While this is extremely beneficial in the long run (more muscle means a higher metabolism), it can drive you crazy in the short run because your scale may not be moving downward even though you are losing body fat. The muscle you are adding is masking the fat you are losing.

You may also be adding muscle if you have just begun exercising or if you recently increased the amount of exercise you are doing. (Many slow losers exercise to accelerate their weight loss and to improve their overall health and fitness.) In the first few days and weeks of exercising, we can add muscle quickly, especially if we have not exercised recently. The combination of increased exercise and increased protein in the diet can increase lean body mass fairly quickly.

In the long term, adding muscle is extremely beneficial in that it takes more energy for our bodies to maintain muscle than it does to maintain fat. It takes approximately 35 to 50 calories a day to maintain a pound of muscle, while it takes only 2 to 3 calories a day to maintain a pound of fat. This is a huge difference. Therefore, adding muscle increases our resting metabolism—that is, the number of calories we burn at rest. While raising our metabolism is always a welcome development, we are challenged in the short term when our scales refuse to budge. Because the added muscle masks the fat loss that is occurring at the same time, our scales are likely to remain the same or even show a slight increase. If we incorrectly assume the stuck scale is evidence the diet is not working, we may become needlessly discouraged. But if we understand that the new muscle weighs more than the fat it replaced, we are much more likely to be patient and allow some time for our bodies to adjust. The fat loss will show on our scales later.

Nori is a great example of how the effects of increased protein intake and increased exercise add muscle and mask fat loss. At the beginning of her low carbohydrate diet, she went through a period in which she believed her weight loss was too slow. She says she was frustrated because she was following the plan faithfully, was drinking plenty of water, and was walking 2.5 miles several times a week, yet her scale refused to move. Nori quickly learned from her peers that she should consider the impact of her previous eating habits on her current rate of weight loss. Before she began her reduced carbohydrate diet, she was on a very strict, very low calorie, and very low fat diet that allowed only 3 ounces of meat or fish per day. She also ate very little protein. Now she understood that adding exercise and increasing her protein intake was allowing her body to build muscle. This new muscle was making it appear as though her weight loss was slow, when in fact, her fat loss was simply hidden *on the scale* by her increased muscle mass. However, although her fat loss was hidden on the scale, it was not hidden from her sight. When she looked in the mirror, her eyes confirmed that she was losing fat while adding muscle. Not only did she see that her legs were becoming much stronger, she noticed that they were becoming much more defined as the muscle was added and the fat was subtracted.

Other evidence that muscle growth masks fat loss is that while the scale reading remains the same, or perhaps even shows a slight increase, *body size decreases*. Many reduced carbohydrate dieters report that although they have gotten back down to the garment size they used to wear, they weigh more than they did when they wore the size the first time because they have more muscle. (This is true even when the recent trend to "vanity size" clothing is taken into account.) They also report that their bodies are shaped differently than before and are much firmer because of the increased muscle. Rachel describes this effect as being much "denser" than she was when she previously wore the same clothes. She says she now feels much "smaller for her weight." Dominick also noticed this pattern and was puzzled by the changes. He questioned his fellow dieters whether his reaction to the diet was typical, since he had not lost any weight according to the scale, yet found his clothes "hanging off" him. "Has this happened to anyone else?" he asked.

Voice of Low Carb Experience

If you previously were a low fat dieter and have recently increased your protein intake or exercise level, you should expect little or no weight loss to show *in the short term* according to the scale, but a decrease in size to occur *in the intermediate to long term*. Without an understanding that your new muscle is masking your body fat loss, you might mistakenly conclude that your diet is not working for you. Your key to success in this situation is to be patient.

The best advice from the seasoned low carbohydrate dieters is: Do not be as concerned with your scale weight as with your body size. In fact, they say, decreased body size should always be celebrated regardless of your scale's feedback. Ask yourself this question: Do I prefer to be lighter or smaller? While these two dimensions of weight loss are interrelated, they are not interchangeable. When muscle is added, it is possible to be smaller without being lighter. Being smaller is much better because muscle is always much more attractive (regardless of its irritating effect on your scale). You should also remind yourself that you are improving your level of fitness, overall health, and metabolism rate by adding muscle. So, if your scale is not moving downward but your body size is, you are losing body fat. It is time to cheer!

The Scale Does Not Tell the Whole Story

Many of us have supernatural beings that dwell in our homes. They are small and silent, but they have a commanding, eerie effect over us nonetheless. They take the form of a common bathroom scale, but like something out of a science fiction movie, they have a mystical, unexplainable grip on us. Each morning, when we rise, the first thing we do is head straight for them with glazed looks in our eyes. If our children or spouses get in our way, we ignore them. We rid ourselves of all matter that may have even the slightest impact on our weight. We strip naked.

We remove all our jewelry, even our glasses. We blow our nose. We trim our nails. We remove the lint from our belly buttons. We exhale air. Then we step on them. They give us a code—a number. And this number sets the whole tone of the day for us. This could be a happy day or it could be a dark day. We know in our hearts that this is ridiculous. We know that they should not have such great power over us. Yet we become slaves to them nonetheless. A part of us hates the sight of them, but we are oddly drawn to them, sometimes several times a day. Rationally, we cannot explain how they can control our lives, but emotionally, we must face it—we are addicted to them.

Then one day, we learn that our scales are not without fault. They have a significant shortcoming in that they measure only our *overall* weight. They do not differentiate body fat from water weight or fluctuating glycogen, and do not take into account the time of day. For many of us, once we realize this weakness, our scales lose their power over us (well, most of it anyway). They once again become simple household appliances—just scales without any magical abilities whatsoever.

Water Retention Masks Fat Loss

In addition to an inability to measure muscle and body fat composition, scales do not give us accurate information about our bodies' daily fluctuations in water content. Water is a very heavy substance that makes up about 50 to 60 percent of our total body mass. In healthcare, professionals have an expression that serves as a rule of thumb about the weight of water: *A pint is a pound the world around.* This means that a pint of water weighs approximately 1 pound. To put this in perspective, 1 pint is 2 cups of fluid. So, for every 2 cups of fluid we drink or discharge, we gain or lose 1 pound of weight according to the scale.

Because water is so heavy, daily fluctuations have big impacts on our scale weights. Our bodies have an amazing ability to constantly adjust our body fluid levels. Therefore, the amount of water we retain can fluctuate by 5 pounds or more each day. In fact, most medical professionals consider a daily fluctuation of up to 3 pounds to be normal.

There are several reasons our bodies' water levels fluctuate. When we increase our amount of exercise, our muscles react by retaining blood and other fluids for the increased nourishment they require to grow. Therefore, one consequence of increased exercise is increased fluid retention by our muscles. Other factors that have strong influences on how much water our bodies hold are how much we sweat, how much sodium we ingest, and how much water we drink. For example, working outside for a day, especially in a hot, dry climate, will cause your body to sweat. Unless you drink enough water to replace the lost fluids, you will likely show a loss on the scale at the end of the day. This loss is temporary, however, because when you drink water to replenish lost fluids, your scale weight once again rises.

Hormones can also have a pronounced effect on how much water our bodies retain, especially for women. While nearly all women retain at least a modest amount of water just before the onset of menstruation, some women can gain 3 to 5 pounds or more. It is very common for this water weight to disappear within a day or two after the beginning of menstruation, but until it does, it will mask any fat loss that occurs at the same time.

The amount of sodium we eat also has a big impact on the amount of water we retain. This topic is discussed in more detail in Chapter 3, but it should be said here that sodium and water go hand in hand. Increased sodium intake causes excess water retention, unless you flush out the excess sodium by drinking a lot of water.

What this means for us is that our scale weight can change by as much as 3 pounds from day to day *regardless of the changes in our body fat stores*. For example, a woman may lose 1 pound of body fat in one week but have a normal water fluctuation that adds 2 pounds of water. Her scale weight temporarily rises by 1 pound, although she lost 1 pound of fat. The additional water is simply masking the fat she lost.

Fluctuating Glycogen Changes the Scale

If growing muscles and shifting water levels were not enough to prove the scale lies, fluctuating stores of glycogen can also confuse the picture. Our bodies have a remarkable ability to take excess glucose from our blood and store it in the liver and muscles in the form of a temporary fuel known as glycogen. Glycogen is stored in these tissues to make it readily available in case the body needs it as a quick source of energy. If the glycogen is not needed (because more carbohydrate is ingested), it is converted to body fat. In this way, glycogen is the temporary storage form of glucose before it becomes body fat. Depending on your daily food intake and activity level, your glycogen stores move up or down from day to day. For people who are on ketogenic diets, the glycogen stores tend to be very low or depleted, which allows the process of ketosis to begin. For people who are not on ketogenic diets, the glycogen stores are much more likely to fluctuate.

For example, a man may put in a strenuous day of exercise. During the course of the day, his body uses his temporary glycogen stores for energy, so when he steps on his scale, he finds that he weighs 2 pounds less than he did before he began the exercise. However, after eating a meal containing carbohydrate, his glycogen stores are quickly restored and the 2 pounds of scale weight return. In this example, the man's body fat stores were unchanged, although his scale weight fluctuated by 2 pounds.

The Time of Day Affects the Scale

The time of day you step on the scale can also significantly influence your scale weight. Most of us are the lightest first thing in the morning. One of the reasons for this is that our kidneys were working all night to remove water while we were not drinking fluids. A second reason is that as we breathe, a small amount of moisture is lost with each exhalation. The combined effects of losing water through urination and moisture through breathing can have a significant impact on our weight in the morning. It is simply because more fluid left the body than came in. As mentioned previously, water is heavy (1 pound per pint), so losing just 2 cups of fluid overnight can cause our scale weight to go down by 1 pound.

We also tend to be the lightest in the morning because our stomachs are empty. It is surprising how often people overlook this simple fact and become frustrated over their weight not falling throughout the day. It should be rather obvious that the weight of the food and fluids we take in during the day causes the scale to fluctuate.

Take Your Measurements

As you can see, merely stepping on the scale will not tell you whether you have lost fat. It will not tell you how much fat you have lost or gained, how much muscle you have lost or gained, how much glycogen you have depleted or replenished, or how much water you have retained. While there are no methods for quickly measuring all these factors at once (short of the technology found on the starship *Enterprise*), there are better ways to gauge fat loss than just stepping on the scale.

The easiest, cheapest, and most common approach is to use a simple, garden-variety tape measure. While nearly all successful reduced carbohydrate dieters recommend that we take our measurements in addition to weighing ourselves, many go even further and recommend that we replace our scales with tape measures. Throw the rascals out. In fact, a rebellious group of female dieters formed a club known as the "SAFF Club," with SAFF standing for Scales Are For Fishes. These ladies refuse to be slaves to the scale and rely only upon the direct feedback their bodies give them, such as body measurements and the fit of their clothes. Their philosophy is that it is more important to be *smaller,* not *lighter,* and the scale will not tell us that. These ladies find the daily fluctuations that occur as a result of factors that have little to do with actual fat loss cause too much angst for them. One of the members says that whether her weight was up or down, she found that getting on the scale triggered her to overeat. If her weight was down, she would think, "Great, I lost some weight; I think I'll reward myself with a treat." If her weight was up, she would think, "Darn, I'm having a bad day already; I think I'll comfort myself with a treat." Either way, she found herself in a daily battle with her scale and her psyche. Once she stopped weighing herself, her weight loss progressed with much less anxiety. Now her philosophy is that she does not care what she weighs; her goal is to wear her old size 10 jeans.

Still, for some of us, it is too much to give up our beloved scales altogether. Many people use a method recommended in *The Carbohydrate Addict's Diet.* They weigh themselves each day and use their daily weights to calculate an average for the week. For example, if a man weighs himself five times during a week and finds his weight to be 195, 197, 197, 195, and 196 pounds, he would average these figures to arrive at a mean of 196 pounds for the week. This weekly average of 196 pounds becomes the point of comparison for tracking and trending. Even with this method, however, many people find it useful to use tape measurements to give themselves another way to track their progress.

The reason the tape measure is such a valuable tool in detecting the fat loss the scale ignores is that muscle weighs more than fat, but *it takes up less space.* New muscle registers as a gain on the scale, but it shows up as a loss with the tape measure. We all find it very motivating and encouraging to discover that we lost inches, especially when our scales are refusing to budge. If we relied solely on our scales, we might mistakenly believe that our diets were not working when in fact we were losing body fat and our body size was decreasing.

Carmen is a great example of the benefit of taking measurements. She began reduced carbohydrate dieting five months before she began an aerobics class. She expected the aerobics class to accelerate her weight loss, but it did not happen. Instead, according to the scale, her weight loss slowed. At first, she was concerned she was in a stall. However, after she measured her dimensions and her body fat percentage, she reevaluated her progress. She was delighted to find that she was most decidedly *not* in a stall. In fact, quite the opposite was true: Her "inches were dropping like flies." She also noticed that her body shape was changing and she looked much more defined. Simply measuring herself allowed her to see that she was losing *body fat*, although the scale was not moving.

Popular areas to measure are the upper arms, bust, waist, hips, and thighs. To be as consistent as possible, the best time of day to measure is first thing in the morning, before eating any food or drinking any fluids. Generally, measurements should be taken no more than once a month because they, too, can fluctuate daily, especially in women. If you are a woman who has menstrual cycles, it is best to measure yourself at the same point in your cycle every month to ensure consistency. One recommended approach is to measure the first thing in the morning following the last day of your period, a time when fluid retention is less troublesome. Because muscles that have recently been stimulated with new or increased exercise will temporarily retain blood and other fluids, it is best to take measurements before an exercise regime is started or increased. After you begin exercising, remember that your measurements will likely show a brief, temporary increase in size until your muscles adjust and the fluid they hold is released.

For people who do not wish to track their measurements in such a formal fashion, a simpler approach is to select a non-stretch article of clothing to serve as a reference for decreasing size. This article of clothing is commonly known as the "reference jeans" to reflect the tendency of people to choose a pair of jeans that were once worn comfortably but are now too small. Belts are also popular choices, especially among men, who tend to gain the majority of their weight around their midsections. The improved comfort and enhanced fit of the reference clothing provides motivation for these folks when the scale is stubborn. Getting into, and actually zipping, a pair of reference jeans is often a festive occasion for reduced carbohydrate dieters—even if the jeans are still too tight to wear in public.

However, there is one irritating aspect of using clothes to serve as the reference in measuring your success: vanity sizing. In response to our nation's growing girth, clothing manufacturers have begun a practice of downsizing clothes. An example of vanity sizing is when a manufacturer places a size 10 label on articles of clothing that were previously considered size 12. Another vanity sizing practice is to design clothing with much more room, such as "relaxed fit" or "loose fit" jeans.

While upscale clothing designers and manufacturers have long practiced vanity sizing, it has become mainstream in recent years. What it means for us is that we may dream of wearing the same size 10 we wore in our youth, but the size 10 we buy today is a larger article of clothing. This shift to bigger sizes has blurred the picture for many of us. Some dieters who are quite irritated by the practice of vanity sizing have sought out jeans at vintage clothing stores that are true to the size of their youth. Pack rats may actually still own the jeans they wore 20 years ago.

Measure Your Body Fat

For those of us who are technically inclined, measuring and tracking our percentage of body fat is also a great gauge of fat loss when the scale is moving slower than we would like. While this measurement involves the use of technology that can sometimes be expensive, it is becoming more accessible and less costly with the production of measuring devices designed for home use. One very popular device is a scale that has a body fat analyzer incorporated into it. This device gives us our weight and body fat percentage each time we step on it. Other smaller, hand-held units are available at department stores. Many health clubs and physician offices offer body fat analysis using more sophisticated and accurate devices and methods. Like tape measurements, body fat percentage measurements should be taken no more than once a month, since the measurements can fluctuate significantly from day to day.

Dalton is a long-term low carbohydrate dieter who much prefers to track his body fat percentage rather than his scale weight. He regularly encourages others to have their body fat percentage measured by a professional at the beginning of their diet and to track it as a measure of their progress. He often cites his personal experience as an example of how it pays off. His first body fat measurement revealed that his body composition was approximately 38 percent fat, a figure well above the recommended range for men. When he was retested after four months of low carbohydrate dieting, his percentage of body fat had dropped to 25 percent, and at seven months, it was down to 21 percent! He found the last analysis to be even more interesting, as it revealed that he had lost 50 pounds of fat but had *gained 7 pounds of muscle!* He says this helps explain why he weighs more now than he did when he wore the same pants several years ago. He believes that if he had only weighed himself on the scale, rather than also measuring his body fat, he would not have been nearly as satisfied with his progress.

Visualize Your Progress

The last—and some say the best—way to gauge your success is to use your eyes. How do you look? Is your face thinner? Do your clothes fit better? Is your shape changing? Do you look more muscular? Even when the scale is slow to move, the loss of body fat can be seen. Tawanna says that when she met a group of friends for drinks one evening, they refused to believe that she had lost only 8 pounds. Because she had been exercising regularly, her shape and posture had changed so much that it appeared she had lost much more.

Voice of Low Carb Experience

One of the keys to success is to consider *all* the indicators of fat loss, not just your scale weight, when you are assessing your weight loss progress. If you can afford it, have your body fat percentage analyzed. At a minimum, get a tape measure and a reliable article of reference clothing and use them. By tracking your measurements and body fat percentage in addition to your scale weight, you decrease the chances that you will mistakenly believe your fat loss is too slow. And as a side benefit, your scale may lose its hold over you and become just a scale once again.

That Time of the Month

Women have long noticed that men lose weight much more quickly and easily than they do, and it is a frequent topic of discussion among them. The most common theory of why this occurs is that male bodies are composed of a higher percentage of muscle than are female bodies. Men's resting metabolism is higher; they burn more calories at rest and, therefore, lose more weight. While this is a valid theory, women have long believed that it does not quite tell the whole story.

Women in their childbearing years are particularly challenged with uneven weight loss because of their monthly menstrual cycle. Every month, they can look forward to a couple of weeks of relatively easy weight loss. That's the good news. The challenge is that these two weeks of normal weight loss are usually followed by two weeks of slowed or nonexistent weight loss. Ladies often politely refer to this time of decreased weight loss as a visit from TOM, an acronym for that "Time Of the Month." TOM is held in almost as much contempt by women as the Carbo Witch. Under the heading of "life is not fair," women spend a great deal of time discussing the irritating effects of their visits from TOM.

The first two weeks of the cycle (the time between the first day of menstruation and the point of ovulation) are a time of relative ease in losing weight. Carbohydrate cravings are usually in check, and hunger is not a daily battle. Women who are on ketogenic diets report that ketosis is relatively painless to achieve and to maintain. For many, all of the weight loss they are able to document, by scale or by tape measure, occurs during this time.

The second two weeks (the time from the point of ovulation to the first day of menstruation) can be quite a different story. Weight loss during this time becomes slow or, worse, virtually stops until menstruation returns. Many women find their ketosis levels decrease sharply or disappear altogether even though they made no changes in their diet or activity. To make this time even more of a challenge, they experience increased hunger and, worst of all, increased carbohydrate cravings. This is a time when chocolate bars become as attractive as fine jewelry. Some women say it feels as though they take one step forward and two steps backward.

Bernadette warned her friends to expect this pattern. She awoke one morning to find herself completely out of ketosis although she had been "doing nothing different."

She was totally puzzled over what she could have eaten that ended her ketosis, so decided to do some research. She discovered that it is common for premenstrual women to go out of ketosis, and she shared her newfound revelation with her friends (in case anyone else was headed to the pantry out of frustration).

There is a silver lining to this dark cloud. If premenstrual women can stick to the plan and keep to their carbohydrate intake goals despite their increased hunger and sugar cravings, they will likely be rewarded with a splendid little whoosh immediately after starting their period. Many women say that their goal during this second two-week time period is simply to maintain their weight, as they are confident their body will give up the fat once menstruation begins. Louisa demonstrated the joy that many women feel once TOM departs from his monthly visit. Just one day after her period ended, she found herself in a much better mood after waking to find a 2-pound whoosh overnight. Not only was this whoosh a great relief for her, but she could also look forward to the next two weeks as a time in which weight loss would be much easier.

To further complicate matters, however, some women report changes in their usual menstrual cycles when they begin a low carbohydrate diet. These changes may be in the frequency, duration, or amount of flow. If a woman experiences changes in the timing or frequency of menstruation, she may have difficulty determining exactly where she is in her cycle. She may not be sure if she is simply experiencing a normal, expected delay in weight loss related to her cycle. However, over several months, most women find that their menstrual cycles once again "even out," and they eventually learn what to expect in each phase of their cycle. Until then, however, they may be frustrated with their rate of loss.

A woman's ability to lose weight can also be complicated if she has had a partial hysterectomy—that is, a hysterectomy in which the ovaries are left intact. In this circumstance, the woman is still producing the hormones related to menstrual cycles, but she does not have the menstrual flow that allows her to track where she is in the hormone cycle. To further complicate matters for women, hormone replacement therapy and birth control pills are other factors that are believed to slow weight loss.

Voice of Low Carb Experience

Sadly, the ladies must accept that this frustrating weight loss pattern is a direct result of Mother Nature and is largely out of their control. But do not give up. Successful women have developed strategies for dealing with the effects of their menstrual cycles.

First, get to know your cycle and its effect on your weight loss. If you are on a ketogenic diet, chart your ketosis each day, at the same time of the day, usually in the morning. If you are not on a ketogenic diet, use your scale and body measurements to track your rate of loss during the two distinct phases of your cycle. For some, a pattern may readily reveal itself, while for others, it may take several months before a discernible pattern begins to emerge.

If your cycle changed recently or if you had a hysterectomy and your ovaries were left intact, you can take your body temperature with a glass thermometer the first thing in the morning each day to determine exactly when you are ovulating. At the time of ovulation, your body temperature will rise, usually about 1°F. This change in body temperature will last until you begin menstruating. About 24 hours before the onset of your period, your body temperature usually will fall back down about 1°F.

The best advice given to women experiencing slow weight loss as a result of their menstrual cycles is not to give in to the increased carbohydrate cravings that occur between ovulation and menstruation. If you can stick with the plan during this time, you are much more likely to be rewarded with a whoosh when your period begins. To fight increased hunger, increase your intake of low carbohydrate foods. Allowing your hunger to go unchecked may be counterproductive because it will increase your vulnerability to carbohydrate cravings. If you give in and eat carbohydrate, you risk a stall (at best) and an actual weight gain (at worst). Lastly, if you are beginning a reduced carbohydrate diet anew or beginning a diet for the first time, try to time your first diet day to fall within the first few days of your menstrual cycle. This step will increase your chances of success, as this is the time during which cravings and hunger are less of a challenge. Starting or restarting a diet in the second half of your menstrual cycle will make your progress much more difficult.

So now that you know the most common patterns of weight loss that people experience while they are losing weight on reduced carbohydrate diets, you will be able to accurately assess your degree of success. If you find yourself in the unfortunate position of feeling frustrated with your rate of weight loss, review these patterns first to be sure that you are not simply experiencing a normal, expected period of slowed weight loss that all of us face at one time or another. If you are, be patient, and all will be well in due time.

However, if you find that your rate of weight loss does not fit one of these patterns or is much slower than that of most reduced carbohydrate dieters (less than one to two pounds per week), you may be inadvertently experiencing one or more stumbling blocks that are slowing your progress. The next chapter looks at the most common factors that are widely believed to slow weight loss and offers advice on what you can do about them.

3
Avoid the Stumbling Blocks

A common expression used by Internet support group participants when they are giving advice is "YMMV," an acronym for "Your Mileage May Vary." This expression means that each of us differs in our reactions to reduced carbohydrate dieting and while certain factors are stumbling blocks for some of us, they have little or no effect on others. The factors discussed in this chapter are the ones blamed most often by seasoned low carbohydrate dieters for slowing weight loss. Two of them, hidden carbohydrate and too many calories, are nearly universal in their effects and touch nearly every reduced carbohydrate dieter at one time or another. The others, however, may affect you or maybe not: YMMV.

Too Much Carbohydrate

For nearly all of us, the amount of weight we lose on reduced carbohydrate diets is directly related to the amount and type of carbohydrate we eat. When we closely adhere to our reduced carbohydrate diet plan and eat less carbohydrate (especially less refined carbohydrate), we lose more weight and lose it more quickly. When we indulge ourselves and eat more carbohydrate (particularly more refined carbohydrate), we lose less weight and lose it more slowly. If we go overboard and eat too much carbohydrate, we experience stalls and plateaus or, even worse, we gain weight. In fact, reduced carbohydrate dieters and experts alike widely believe that eating too much carbohydrate, particularly too much simple carbohydrate, is the most common reason for limited success on the reduced carbohydrate diet plans.

Refined Versus Natural Carbohydrate Sources

Many new low carbohydrate dieters who are frustrated with their slow rate of weight loss have not yet learned what the seasoned low carbohydrate dieters already know: The source of the carbohydrate we eat makes a big difference in our rate of weight loss. While several reduced carbohydrate diet book authors place a great deal of emphasis on the differences in the sources of carbohydrate, some of them mention it only briefly. These authors inadvertently give us an inaccurate impression that the source of the carbohydrate we eat does not matter as long as we keep our total carbohydrate intake low. Therefore, some new reduced carbohydrate dieters may unwittingly slow their weight loss by eating the wrong type of carbohydrate even though they keep their total carbohydrate intake down.

The truth is that when it comes to triggering insulin releases and losing weight, all sources of carbohydrate are not created equal. There are very important differences in "fattening power" between simple, refined carbohydrate sources and complex, natural carbohydrate sources. Simple, refined carbohydrate wreaks havoc because it causes much higher blood glucose levels and greater insulin releases than do complex, unrefined sources. And as we know, large, sudden insulin releases slow weight loss.

Foods made of simple, refined carbohydrate break down easily in the stomach and intestines and enter the bloodstream quickly. As a result, the glucose in the blood quickly rises to a level high enough to prompt an immediate large release of insulin, which slows weight loss. On the other hand, foods made of complex, natural carbohydrate (particularly foods with high fiber contents) do not cause such sudden rises in blood glucose levels. Because fiber slows digestion, the carbohydrate in these foods enters our blood much more slowly. Less insulin is produced in response and weight loss proceeds. The cold, harsh reality is that a piece of chocolate with 30 grams of refined carbohydrate will cause higher glucose levels, greater insulin releases, and slower weight loss than broccoli with 30 grams of carbohydrate. While this is hardly joyful news for any of us, the upside is that simply shifting from eating refined foods to more unprocessed, unrefined foods can have a significant impact on your rate of weight loss. (For more information about preferred carbohydrate sources, see Chapter 4.)

Hidden Carbohydrate

Hidden carbohydrate is one of the primary reasons we take in too much carbohydrate, and we are all victims of it at one time or another. Hidden carbohydrate is carbohydrate that is not immediately obvious in products, even by reading the Nutritional Facts label. This is because the guidelines governing food labels allow manufacturers to list the carbohydrate content of a food as 0 grams if the actual count is less than 1 gram per serving. The thought is that a count of less than 1 gram is of no consequence in the diet, so accuracy at this level is not necessary. While most reduced carbohydrate dieters have come to think of a food with 0 grams of carbohydrate (according to the Nutrition Facts label) as one they can eat in unlimited amounts, the truth is that nearly all foods have some carbohydrate in them and these small hidden amounts can really add up. There are very few foods that are truly carbohydrate-free. To make matters worse, the carbohydrate hidden in products is almost always a refined carbohydrate, most often simple sugar.

The best way to uncover the hidden carbohydrate in a food is to analyze the counts on its nutritional label to see if they add up. The simplest method is to use the rounded values of 9 calories per gram of fat, 4 calories per gram of protein, and 4 calories per gram of carbohydrate to calculate the total calories. If the nutritional values do not add up to the total calories figure on the label, the manufacturer probably rounded down the true carbohydrate content. Some manufacturers just remove the fiber count from the total carbohydrate count. Both of these practices allow the total carbohydrate figure to appear lower.

For example, the nutritional label in Figure 3.1 was on a package of heavy whipping cream I purchased at my local grocery store. As is true with most brands of cream, the Nutrition Facts label on this product listed the carbohydrate count as 0 grams. However, close examination of the label shows why cream is often cited as an example of how a product may contain carbohydrate that is not included on the label.

First, the serving size is small—only 1 tablespoon—and the carbohydrate count is 0 grams. This combination alone should raise our suspicions. This very small serving size may have resulted in a carbohydrate count that was less than 1 gram, thereby allowing the manufacturer to round

Nutrition Facts

Serving Size 1 Tbsp (15 ml)
Servings Per Container 16

Amount Per Serving	
Calories 50	**Calories from Fat** 45

	% Daily Value*
Total Fat 5g	8%
Saturated Fat 4g	18%
Cholesterol 20mg	7%
Sodium 5mg	0%
Total Carbohydrate 0g	0%
Dietary Fiber 0g	0%
Sugars 0g	
Protein 0g	Not a significant source of protein

Vitamin A	4%	Vitamin C	0%
Calcium	0%	Iron	0%

*Percent Daily Values are based on a 2,000 calorie diet.

INGREDIENTS: CREAM, MONO- AND
DIGLYCERIDES, POLYSORBATE 80 AND
CARRAGEENAN.

Figure 3.1. The very small serving size used on this label has brought the carbohydrate count of this product down to less than 1 gram, allowing the manufacturer to round it down to 0 grams.

it down to 0 grams. Another clue is that the ingredient list includes items other than cream, which may add carbohydrate.

The next step is to calculate the total calories based upon the nutritional information given on the label. The label lists 5 grams of fat. Since each gram of fat contributes 9 calories, the fat in the product accounts for 45 of the 50 total calories given on the label. The protein content is given as 0 grams; therefore, 5 calories are missing in that they are not accounted for on the label. Since each gram of carbohydrate contributes 4 calories, we can estimate that this product may have as much as 1.25 grams of hid-

den carbohydrate per 1-tablespoon serving (5 missing calories divided by 4 calories per gram of carbohydrate
equals 1.25 grams of carbohydrate).

The next step is to verify the nutritional content of
cream with a source independent of the manufacturer. A
quick check of the USDA database reveals that our estimate of 1.25 grams of carbohydrate is higher than the 0.4
gram of carbohydrate per tablespoon (6.6 grams per cup)
given by the USDA. This difference can be partially explained by the fact that the USDA also gives a protein
value of 0.3 gram that this manufacturer rounded down to
0 grams. By taking the USDA's value of 0.3 gram of protein
into consideration, we can estimate that approximately 1.2
calories in this product are due to its protein content.
Therefore, fat and protein contribute approximately 46
calories to the total, leaving a difference of 4 calories. By
dividing the 4 missing calories by 4 calories per gram of
carbohydrate, we arrive at a new estimate of 1 gram of carbohydrate per tablespoon. While this estimate remains
higher than the USDA's figure of 0.4 gram of carbohydrate, the difference can be partially explained by the fact
that this product is not pure cream—it has three additional
ingredients that may contribute carbohydrate to the product.

As a second example, I found the label in Figure 3.2 at-
tached to a very popular drink mix. It is a glaring example
of hidden carbohydrate, since the nutritional values for
carbohydrate, fat, and protein are all listed as 0 grams, yet
the calorie count for an 8-ounce serving is 5 calories.

Since we know that the only sources of calories in our
diet are the three macronutrients (carbohydrate, fat, and
protein), it is not possible for the values of all three of
these to be zero if the product contains calories. Therefore, we should immediately suspect hidden carbohydrate.
Reviewing the ingredient list reveals the product contains

Nutrition Facts

Serving Size 1/8 tub (1.7g)
(Makes 8 fl oz)
Servings 32

Amount Per Serving	
Calories 5	

	% DV*
Total Fat 0g	0%
Sodium 0mg	0%
Total Carbohydrate 0g	0%
Dietary Fiber 0g	0%
Sugars 0g	
Protein 0g	

Not a significant source of calories from Fat, Saturated Fat, Cholesterol, Dietary Fiber, Vitamin A, Vitamin C, Calcium, and Iron

*Percent Daily Values (DV) are based on a 2,000 calorie diet.

INGREDIENTS: Citric Acid (Provides Tartness), Potassium Citrate (Controls Acidity), Aspartame (Sweetener), Maltodextrin (From Corn), Magnesium Oxide (Prevents Caking), Natural Flavor, Acesulfame Potassium, Artificial Color, Red 40 Lake, Yellow 6, BHA (Preserves Freshness).

Figure 3.2. The 5 calories per serving on this label indicate that something is wrong with the 0-gram counts given for the total fat, total carbohydrate, and protein contents of this product.

maltodextrin, a disguised sugar that is a source of carbohydrate (see page 152). We can estimate that this product has approximately 1.25 grams of carbohydrate per 8-ounce serving by dividing the 5 calories by the 4 calories provided by each gram of carbohydrate.

Coffee is another example. Many people assume that plain black coffee is carbohydrate-free, when in fact, with or without caffeine, coffee has approximately 1 gram of carbohydrate per cup. Some of the flavored coffees that are popular at specialty coffee shops often have even more carbohydrate. For those dieters who drink considerable amounts of coffee, especially if they add artificial sweeteners and cream, the extra carbohydrate can really add up. Sugar-free breath mints and sugar-free gums are other common sources of hidden carbohydrate to the tune of approximately 2 grams per stick. It may sound as though these hidden amounts of carbohydrate are trivial, but many people find that they must be concerned with them anyway, especially if they are on ketogenic diets, if their weight loss is very slow, or they become stuck in a plateau.

The greatest benefit of nutritional label analysis is that it allows us to make more informed choices about which foods we should eliminate from our diet and which foods we can include. For example, Kurt found that his favorite brand of sour cream and onion pork rinds contained dextrose even though the carbohydrate content was listed as 0 grams. His reaction was one of disappointment because he was going to have to "toss them in the trash," as he put it. Had he performed an analysis, he might have found that they contained few enough grams of carbohydrate that he could have fit a serving or two into his diet.

Overlooked Carbohydrate

In addition to watching for carbohydrate that is hidden from our sight, we also need to be careful that we don't simply overlook some not-so-obvious sources of carbohydrate. This carbohydrate is referred to as "overlooked carbohydrate" rather than "hidden carbohydrate" because it is clearly listed on food labels and in nutrition counters, but for a variety of reasons is simply overlooked. For example, while meat generally is carbohydrate-free, some varieties, such as deli-style meats, cured meats, and sausages, contain carbohydrate that we may fail to notice.

For example, after Darcy learned about overlooked carbohydrate in herbs and seasonings, she began to investigate the carbohydrate count of the seasonings she used in a homemade salad dressing that she ate nearly every day. Her son mentioned to her that the balsamic vinegar she used as a base for the salad dressing tasted sweet to him, so she reviewed its label closely. She was shocked to learn that it contained 6 grams of carbohydrate *per tablespoon*. This meant that she was eating approximately 30 to 36 grams of carbohydrate per day that she had simply overlooked. The carbohydrate count was clearly printed on the label, but she did not read the label because she had simply assumed that all vinegars were carbohydrate-free.

Some of the most frequently overlooked sources of carbohydrate are:

- *Artificial sweeteners.* Most powdered artificial sweeteners, including aspartame, saccharin, acesulfame-k, and sucralose, have approximately 1 gram of carbohydrate per small individual serving packet (1-teaspoon size).
- *Cheese.* Cheese is commonly viewed as carbohydrate-free, when in fact, most varieties actually contain approximately 1 gram of carbohydrate per ounce.
- *Eggs.* Eggs are also considered carbohydrate-free. In reality, they contain approximately 0.6 to 1.0 gram of carbohydrate, depending upon their size.
- *Onions.* Because of our lifetime of experience with low fat diets, many of us have become accustomed to eating onions without concern. However, onions are a significant source of carbohydrate, containing 12 to 14 grams per cup when chopped.
- *"Sugar-free" foods.* Foods labeled "sugar-free" often contain substantial amounts of carbohydrate from fillers and other ingredients. Common examples are breath mints, gum, gelatin, drink mixes, and syrup.

- *Low fat substitutes*. Many popular low fat products have substantial amounts of added sugar. Manufacturers add sugar in an attempt to replace the taste that is lost when the fat is removed. The classic example is salad dressings: Original ranch salad dressing has only about 1 gram of carbohydrate per tablespoon, while its low fat counterpart has three to four times more.

- *Sweet pickles*. While some pickles, such as dill pickles, have little or no carbohydrate, sweet pickles are cured with significant amounts of sugar.

- *Mayonnaise-based salads*. While the main ingredients in most of these salads, such as the chicken and mayonnaise in chicken salad, contain little or no carbohydrate, the other ingredients, such as onions and sweet pickles, can add sizable amounts of carbohydrate.

- *Mayonnaise substitutes*. Many of the popular mayonnaise substitutes, commonly known as sandwich spreads, may look and taste very much like mayonnaise, but they have substantial amounts of sugar. Mayonnaise generally has less than 1 gram of carbohydrate per tablespoon, while sandwich spreads may have up to 4 grams of carbohydrate per tablespoon. This can be particularly hazardous when eating out, as many restaurants use mayonnaise substitutes rather than real mayonnaise in their recipes.

- *Restaurant salad dressings*. Many restaurants have an irritating practice of adding sugar to salad dressings that are otherwise low carbohydrate. For example, most ranch-style salad dressings have approximately 1 gram of carbohydrate per tablespoon. However, the ranch dressing at one of the world's most famous fast-food restaurants has 10 grams of carbohydrate per 2-tablespoon-size packet.

- *Seafood substitutes*. Most seafood has a very low or

nonexistent carbohydrate count, but imitation seafood is a different story. For example, 4 ounces of real crabmeat has a near zero carbohydrate count, while the same amount of imitation crabmeat made from surimi has a carbohydrate count of 10 to 12 grams. Again, you need to be especially watchful in restaurants, which like to use imitation seafood in salads.

- *Non-dairy creamers.* Be wary of those little liquid coffee creamers you get in restaurants. While many are real cream or half and half, both of which have small amounts of carbohydrate, some are cream substitutes that carry a carbohydrate blast. For example, some of the flavored versions contain 5 to 7 grams of carbohydrate each.

- *Fillers.* Fillers hide in prepared dishes and sneak in carbohydrate. The most common example is the bread filler in meatballs and meat loaves. (Many people suggest substituting firm tofu for the bread filler as a great way to cut out the carbohydrate in those dishes.)

- *Condiments.* All those little "add-ons" that spice up our food, such as ketchup (4 grams of carbohydrate per tablespoon), can be a significant source of overlooked carbohydrate. Likewise, barbecue sauce is often surprisingly sugar-laden.

- *Spices and cooking additives.* Believe it or not, adding spices or other ingredients to recipes can add carbohydrate. For example, curry powder has approximately 4 grams of carbohydrate per tablespoon, onion powder has approximately 5 grams of carbohydrate per tablespoon, and garlic powder has approximately 6 grams of carbohydrate per tablespoon.

- *Milk.* New low carbohydrate dieters are often surprised to learn that milk has a significant amount of carbohydrate. Whole, skim, and 2 percent milk have approximately 11.4 grams of carbohydrate per cup. (Many people use a diluted cream mixture of half water and half cream as a substitute for milk in recipes.)

- *Instant tea.* While brewed tea is free of carbohydrate, instant tea is another matter. Many brands of powdered tea mixes use an ingredient known as maltodextrin that adds approximately 1 gram of carbohydrate per 8-ounce glass.

Having your diet analyzed by people who are experienced in reduced carbohydrate dieting may prove helpful in uncovering hidden and overlooked carbohydrate. If you have access to an Internet group, post a sample daily menu under a heading such as "Attention: Carb Detectives" to alert the group participants that you need help. They will review the content of your food diary and offer advice to help you ferret out hidden and overlooked carbohydrate.

This technique worked very well for Veronica. Early in her diet, she began to worry that the diet was not working for her. She was concerned because her weight loss seemed slow even though she was keeping her daily carbohydrate count consistently below 30 grams. Her fellow low carbohydrate dieters immediately suspected hidden and overlooked carbohydrate and asked Veronica to keep a diet journal for a typical day. Table 3.1 shows the foods Veronica ate, the carbohydrate counts she had established, and the actual carbohydrate counts she found by looking up the food in a gram counter. What a difference!

Veronica was shocked to learn through this review that she was overlooking several sources of carbohydrate, most of which came from foods she thought were carbohydrate-free, such as eggs, cheese, kielbasa, lettuce, whipped cream, coffee, cream, artificial sweeteners, and sugar-free

Table 3.1. Veronica's diet journal for a typical day.

Food	Quantity	Estimated carbohydrate count	Actual carbohydrate count
Eggs	3	0	2
Cheese	2 ounces	0	2
Chicken breasts	2	0	0
Pumpkin seeds	1 ounce	4	4
Turkey kielbasa	6 ounces	0	6
Lettuce	2 cups	0	4
Salad dressing	¼ cup	4	4
Broccoli	1 cup	2	2*
Cauliflower	1 cup	3	3*
Green beans	½ cup	2	2*
Sugar-free gelatin	½ cup	0	0
Whipped cream	¼ cup	0	2
Coffee	4 cups	0	4
Cream	4 tablespoons	0	2
Artificial sweeteners	5 packets	0	5
Sugar-free gum	2 pieces	0	4
Totals		15	48

*Figures represent the "digestible carbohydrate" count.

gum. In a typical day, she underestimated her intake by 33 grams of carbohydrate, consuming three times more carbohydrate than she estimated.

Disguised Sugars

The ingredient lists on product packages reveal a wealth of information about the true carbohydrate content of foods, and we should diligently review them on everything we eat. While it can be laborious, reading ingredient lists can really pay off by helping us uncover disguised sugars. Disguised sugars are sources of carbohydrate that may not be immediately obvious by reading product packages. In what seems to be a conspiracy designed to drive reduced carbohydrate dieters and diabetics crazy, disguised sugars are particularly prevalent in so-called sugar-free products.

In the United States, food manufacturers are allowed to label foods as sugar-free if the foods do not contain sucrose, or common table sugar. However, they are allowed to include several other sugars in their sugar-free products as substitutes for the sucrose. Although nutritional experts widely believe that sucrose substitutes are digested more slowly than sucrose, thereby raising blood glucose levels more slowly than sucrose, they are sugars nonetheless and made up of carbohydrate. Therefore, it is very common to find "sugar-free" foods and products that contain significant, sometimes large, amounts of carbohydrate. Fortunately for us, although food producers are allowed to slip these sugars into the products they label as sugar-free, they must include them in the ingredient list and in the carbohydrate and calorie counts. Because of this, they are relatively easy to find—if you know what to look for.

While reading an ingredient list sounds like an uncomplicated task, understanding it well enough to uncover disguised sugars is not always so simple. Disguised sugars often masquerade under complicated technical names, making their unmasking more difficult. For most of us, deciphering these technical names can present a significant challenge in and of itself, but there are clues to guide us if we know how to recognize them. For example, disguised sugars often end in the suffix *ose,* such as glucose, fructose, dextrose, maltose, lactose, xylose, levulose, saccharose, mannose, and sucrose. All of these ingredients are sugars although they may appear to be elements from a chemistry laboratory. Maltodextrin, dextrin, turbinado, and treacle are also disguised sugars that are sources of carbohydrate. Another carbohydrate group, commonly known as "sugar alcohols," is often listed under the names of sorbitol, mannitol, xylitol, dulcitol, isomalt, lactitol, and maltilol. Sugar alcohols are very common in sugar-free candies and snack products. Other simpler, more common sugars that could be lurking in your food are corn syrup, molasses, carob, sorghum, starch, and honey. The presence of these disguised sugars explains why a statement such as "Not a Reduced Calorie Food" is often found on sugar-free products.

For example, Figure 3.3 shows the label from a package of "sugar-free" candies I bought at my local grocery store. Although the phrase "sugar-free" was emblazoned in huge letters on the front of the package, the Nutrition Facts label revealed that the product was far from carbohydrate-free. In fact, a single, very small piece of this candy had 6 grams of carbohydrate, with the designated serving of four small pieces containing 24 grams of carbohydrate.

How can this "sugar-free" product contain so much carbohydrate? The answer lies in the ingredient list and on the Nutrition Facts label, as they tell us this product has a very common disguised sugar —maltitol. Furthermore, since the maltitol is one of the first ingredients on the list, and ingredients are listed in order from the greatest amount to least amount, we can assume that this product contains significant amounts of it. In fact, the Nutrition Facts label gives a value of 22 grams of maltitol in the space where the sugar content is usually provided.

Sylvia learned a painful lesson about believing the "sugar-free" declaration on a box of chocolates. Her coworker offered her a piece of sugar-free chocolate at work. Before Sylvia ate it, she asked her coworker if she was sure it was sugar-free. The coworker showed her the box, which clearly said "sugar-free" on the front. Within a few minutes of eating three of the chocolates, Sylvia had a headache. She was immediately suspicious of the choco-

Nutrition Facts

Serving Size 4 pieces (36g)
Servings Per Container About 3

Amount Per Serving	
Calories 200	**Calories from Fat** 100

	% Daily Value*
Total Fat 11g	17%
Saturated Fat 7g	35%
Cholesterol <5mg	1%
Sodium 10mg	0%
Total Carbohydrate 24g	8%
Dietary Fiber <1g	4%
Maltitol 22g	
Protein 2g Not a significant source of protein	

Vitamin A	0%	Vitamin C	0%
Calcium	0%	Iron	2%

*Percent Daily Values are based on a 2,000 calorie diet.
Your daily values may be higher or lower depending on
your caloric needs.

	Calories:	2,000	2,500
Total Fat	Less than	65g	80g
Sat. Fat	Less than	20g	25g
Cholesterol	Less than	300mg	300mg
Sodium	Less than	2,400mg	2,400mg
Total Carbohydrate		300g	375g
Dietary Fiber		25mg	30g

Calories per gram:
Fat 9 • Carbohydrate 4 • Protein 4

INGREDIENTS: Sugar Free Chocolate (Maltitol),
Cocoa Butter, Chocolate Liquor, Cocoa Powder,
Sodium Caseinate, Milk Fat, Lecithin (Emulsifier),
Acesulfame-k, Salt, Natural and Artificial Flavor,
Lycasin, Maltisorb, Butter, Natural and Artificial
Flavor and Lecithin (An Emulsifier).

Figure 3.3. The Nutrition Facts label and ingredient list of this
"sugar-free" product show that it contains 22 grams
of disguised sugar.

late because she had not experienced any of her usual migraines since beginning her reduced carbohydrate diet. She found the box, read the ingredient list, and discovered it included sugar alcohols and several other ingredients with the *ose* ending, confirming her suspicions that the product contained a significant amount of carbohydrate.

Misleading Labels

As if the legitimate rounding down of real carbohydrate counts and sneaking of sugars into "sugar-free" products is not enough to drive some of us crazy, a further aggravation is when labels are blatantly incorrect or intentionally misleading. Occasionally, the carbohydrate count given on a Nutrition Facts label is so inaccurate, it cannot be explained simply by the rounding down of figures or substitution of sugars. To illustrate this point, Figure 3.4 shows a nutritional label from a bottle of salad dressing I purchased by chance at my local grocery store. I originally purchased this product because it had a low carbohydrate count on the label. However, when I added up the label values at home, I was shocked at the inaccuracy. It is a great example of how products can have seriously misleading labels.

After simply glancing at this Nutrition Facts label in the store, I had assumed that this product was a great carbohydrate bargain. The carbohydrate count was presented as only 1 gram per 2 tablespoons of dressing, or only 0.5 gram of carbohydrate per tablespoon. However, when I tried the dressing at home, it tasted sweet. The sweet taste prompted me to read the ingredient list, which immediately raised my suspicions that the label was inaccurate. The ingredient list included tahini, cider vinegar, lemon juice, garlic, and sesame seeds, all of which contain carbo-

Nutrition Facts	
Serving Size 2 Tbsp (29g)	
Servings Per Container About 8	

Amount Per Serving	
Calories 90	**Calories from Fat** 70
	% Daily Value*
Total Fat 8g	13%
Saturated Fat 1g	6%
Sodium 310mg	13%
Total Carbohydrate 1g	1%
Dietary Fiber 2g	
Sugars 0g	
Protein 0g Not a significant source of protein	

*Percent Daily Values are based on a 2,000 calorie diet. Your daily values may be higher or lower depending on your caloric needs.

INGREDIENTS: Expeller Pressed Canola Oil, Water, Tahini, Cider Vinegar, Shoyu, Lemon Juice, Sea Salt, Garlic, Toasted Sesame Seeds, Parsley, Chives, Xanthan Gum.

Figure 3.4. This Nutrition Facts label and ingredient list from a bottle of "low carb" salad dressing indicate the manufacturer was trying to mislead consumers.

hydrate. Given these ingredients, I concluded that it was unlikely that this product could contain as little as 0.5 gram of carbohydrate per tablespoon.

My next step was to calculate the total calorie count based upon the nutritional information provided on the label. The total fat content was listed as 8 grams per serving. Since fat contains 9 calories per gram, I knew that 72 calories were derived from fat. The protein content was listed as 0 grams per serving; therefore the calories from fat and protein added up to a total of only 72 calories. However, the total calorie figure was listed as 90 calories per serving—a whopping difference of 18 calories. Dividing the 18 "missing" calories by 4 (the number of calories per 1 gram of carbohydrate), I estimated that the product may have actually contained as much as 4.5 grams of carbohydrate per serving, over four and a half times the amount given on the label. The discrepancy between the calories I calculated and the total calories listed on the label could not be explained by the practice of simply rounding down.

Another glaring discrepancy on this label was that the very low carbohydrate count of 1 gram per serving directly contradicted the fiber count of 2 grams per serving. Since the total carbohydrate count is the sum of the fiber count and the sugar count (plus other carbohydrate), it is not possible for the total carbohydrate count to be less than the fiber count. Needless to say, I did not eat the remainder of the dressing.

Unfortunately, inaccurate labels such as this one are all too common. Periodically, news of a product whose label has been found to misrepresent the true carbohydrate count spreads like wildfire among reduced carbohydrate dieters. In fact, some people have been so suspicious of misleading product labels that they funded nutritional analyses by independent laboratories to learn the accurate carbohydrate counts, with surprising results.

One particular story illustrates this point well. Several members of three Internet news groups were suspicious of the carbohydrate count on the label of a brand of low carbohydrate mini-bagels that "tasted too good to be true." The company that baked the bagels claimed they were made of whole-grain wheat fiber. The nutritional counts on the package were listed as 60 calories, 12 grams of carbohydrate, and a whopping 9 grams of fiber per bagel. Because the digestible carbohydrate count was only 3 grams (derived by subtracting the fiber count from the total carbohydrate count), these bagels were very popular among reduced carbohydrate dieters. Many dieters who struggled with bread cravings ate the bagels regularly.

These folks' suspicions were so strong that they pooled their money and paid a substantial fee to an independent, certified laboratory to have a nutritional analysis of the bagels performed. The results were shocking: The total calorie count was 80 calories, the total carbohydrate count was 15 grams, and the fiber count was 7 grams. The digestible carbohydrate content was really 8 grams, or nearly three times greater than the package stated. Needless to say, the news of this analysis sparked anger among the people who regularly ate the bagels.

Months later, the company changed its recipe, and the nutritional values on the labels were changed. The new product was also tested, although it was funded by another person and conducted at a different laboratory. This time, the label values were found to be accurate.

Something similar happened when Kevin became suspicious of a brand of crackers that boasted a very low carbohydrate count of 2.5 grams. Kevin contacted the company that manufactured the crackers asking for verification. The company responded by stating that the label was indeed in error. The true carbohydrate count was 22 grams. The manufacturer placed the blame on the printer, who apparently inserted a decimal point that should not have been included.

Lorraine tells a similar story with an opposite outcome. While shopping at an upscale gourmet grocer, she purchased a large, very expensive bottle of seasoned oil. After learning about hidden carbohydrate and investigating all of the products in her pantry, she was shocked to find that the carbohydrate count of the oil was 5.5 grams per 2 teaspoons. She immediately threw the oil away. When she complained to the manufacturer, she was told that the label was wrong and the carbohydrate count was actually 0 grams.

Voice of Low Carb Experience

Seasoned low carbohydrate dieters have learned through unpleasant (sometimes painful) experiences to do research, research, and more research to learn as much as they can about the foods they eat. You must do the same. Unfortunately, since so many foods contain hidden carbohydrate and disguised sugars, you must become a super sleuth.

Read both the Nutrition Facts label and the ingredient list on all the foods you eat. First, calculate the nutritional values given on the Nutrition Facts label to verify its accuracy. Be very suspicious when the carbohydrate count is given as 0 grams, the serving size is small, or the ingredient list contains sugars or other common sources of carbohydrate, especially if they are among the first ingredients listed. If you find a discrepancy on the label, assume that the food contains hidden carbohydrate. The general rule of thumb is: If there are sugars or other sources of carbohydrate in the ingredient list, there is carbohydrate in the food. You should count at least 0.5 gram of carbohydrate per serving if carbohydrate sources are included in the ingredient list, even if the Nutrition Facts label says 0 grams.

You must also learn to be suspicious of misleading labels, whether the result of deliberate or accidental misrepresentation by the manufacturers. If you are losing weight very slowly, or if you are stuck in a plateau, eliminate all suspicious foods, even if their Nutrition Facts labels add up properly. Rule out foods that look "too good to be true," such as breads, crackers, tortillas, and pastas that boast a low carbohydrate count. Remember the old adage: If it looks too good to be true, it probably is.

Independent resources such as published nutritional counters and the USDA's on-line food database (http://www.nal.usda.gov/fnic/cgi-bin/nut_search.pl) are very helpful in verifying the accuracy of Nutrition Facts labels. They are also essential for looking up foods that do not have Nutrition Facts labels, such as fresh produce. Use your independent source to look up all the foods you eat, even if you are fairly certain they do not contain carbohydrate. Blithely assuming a food does not have much carbohydrate can be a big mistake that adds a significant amount of carbohydrate to your diet.

All seasoned low carbohydrate dieters know that restaurants are virtual minefields when it comes to hidden carbohydrate. However, there are a few resources that can help you. Many chain restaurants, especially fast-food restaurants, have nutritional brochures and web sites that provide the nutritional contents of their dishes. Ask for them and use them. If you can, join an Internet reduced carbohydrate diet group and ask the participants for the carbohydrate count of dishes you cannot find. The experienced carbohydrate detectives who regularly participate in these groups can be great resources.

Although this research may be time-consuming and tedious, it can give you valuable insights into your real carbohydrate intake. By not taking all sources of carbohydrate into consideration, you could be unknowingly consuming significant amounts of carbohydrate. As little as 5 to 10 grams of carbohydrate per day, especially if it is in the form of simple, refined carbohydrate, will probably affect nearly everyone in some way, and the addition of 10 grams of carbohydrate per day can definitely slow weight loss to a snail's pace for some.

Too Little Carbohydrate

A much less frequently mentioned stumbling block is taking in *too little* carbohydrate. Although taking in too little carbohydrate is not often discussed among reduced carbohydrate dieters (we all seem to struggle with the other end of the spectrum), several of the reduced carbohydrate diet book authors strongly believe that taking in too little carbohydrate over long periods of time can ultimately lead to slow weight loss. Their theory is that: a long period of very low carbohydrate intake can cause the body to become more efficient at burning fuel. The result is a sluggish metabolism that slows weight loss. (It is important to note that other reduced carbohydrate diet book authors strongly disagree with this theory.)

Voice of Low Carb Experience

If you have truly been eating a very low level of carbohydrate (with no accidental ingestion of hidden or overlooked carbohydrate) for a long period, usually months, your body may be getting much more efficient at processing carbohydrate and your weight loss may slow in response. You may need to add complex, unrefined sources of carbohydrate to jump-start your weight loss. However, adding carbohydrate should be done slowly and carefully. For example, a common approach is to add no more than 5 grams of complex carbohydrate per day for three days and then maintain that level of intake for about a week to see if it helps.

For people on ketogenic diets, a common approach is to add 5 grams of complex carbohydrate per day until ketosis stops. Then, remove the 5 grams of carbohydrate again to return to ketosis and watch for about a week to see if this rejuvenates your weight loss.

A word of caution: The sources of the additional carbo-hydrate should be vegetables or other appropriate foods, rather than simple sugars such as that tempting box of chocolates.

Calories

For nearly all of us, one of the greatest attractions of reduced carbohydrate dieting is the wonderful freedom from counting calories. Most of us have counted calories for years and have found little, if any, success and, frankly, are bored with it. Several of the best-selling authors know us very well and use this calorie-counting discontent to their marketing advantage. They boldly state "Never Count Calories Again" on their book covers and on their web sites.

For the lucky ones among us, the promise is fulfilled, and counting only grams of carbohydrate works very well. These people never count calories and their weight loss progresses. Others find that they can disregard calories in the early stages of their diet, but must count them later on, especially as they approach their goal weights. They find that without taking calories into consideration, their weight loss slows substantially the lighter they become. Still others find that they must consider calories from the very beginning to be successful. Usually, these people have less to lose, but it can be true for any of us, regardless of our starting weight.

Too Many Calories

Eating too much food is a close second to eating too much carbohydrate as a leading cause of slow weight loss, stalls, and plateaus. Most of the reduced carbohydrate diet book authors state in their books or on their web sites that calories do count *for some of us*. While it is common for a new dieter to mistakenly conclude that reduced carbohydrate diets are all-you-can-eat diets, close inspection of the authors' statements reveals words of caution. For example, two of the authors who state on their web site that you need "never count calories again" state in their book that "you usually do not have to count calories on the program." Nearly all of the reduced carbohydrate diet book authors agree that a person should eat until satisfied, not until stuffed, and because of the satiety of fat and protein, "calories will take care of themselves." The idea is that since fat and protein make us feel much fuller for a longer period of time, we naturally eat less overall and thereby reduce our calorie intake naturally. However, some people find that old habits die hard and, even with the increased satiety of protein and fat, continue to eat more than is necessary. For them, calorie intake is a factor. Among the seasoned reduced carbohydrate dieters and experts alike, there is little doubt that a person will lose more weight, and lose it more quickly, on a 2,000-calorie, 50-gram-carbohydrate diet than on a 3,000-calorie, 50-gram-carbohydrate diet.

For example, Trent discovered the impact of calories on his rate of weight loss. While he understood that his chosen diet was not intended to be calorie driven, he found that his love of red meat was causing his weight to plateau. When his weight loss stopped, he was advised to consider that too many calories might be a cause of his stall. He listened and to his shock discovered that he was eating about 3,500 calories per day. He found that the main contributor to his high calorie count was red meat. When he lowered his overall calorie intake by substituting chicken and fish for the meat, his weight loss resumed.

Although many of us find ourselves under a dark cloud when we realize we must lower our calorie intake to jump-start our weight loss, we also find a bit of a silver lining when we discover our calorie intake can be considerably higher on reduced carbohydrate diets than on our previous low fat diets. For example, Jonas said he tracked his calorie intake for years while eating a low fat diet and found that, to lose weight, he had to keep his calorie count very low. With reduced carbohydrate dieting, he also found he had to watch his calorie intake to lose weight, but was pleased to realize that the total number of calories he could consume and still lose weight was much higher.

Too Much Dairy

Dairy products are treasured by many reduced carbohydrate dieters because they are very low in carbohydrate, yet have a rich taste. The challenge is that many dairy products are also very calorie-dense. Therefore, an over-indulgence in cheese, cream, or cream cheese, for example, can add enough calories to our daily total to slow our weight loss. (Usually, cheese is the culprit.) Since most low carbohydrate treats and desserts are made from dairy products, it can be easy for us to overindulge. Our mistake is that we believe unlimited low carbohydrate treats are acceptable as long as our total carbohydrate count is restricted. What we learn is that our total calorie count can be high enough to slow our weight loss even though our carbohydrate count is low.

For example, Jessica loved her homemade low carbohydrate fudge (made from cream cheese), and she considered it one of the greatest pleasures of reduced carbohydrate living. However, she learned that although she kept her overall carbohydrate count low, the extra calories in the fudge caused her weight loss to stall. Once she limited her intake of the fudge (and other dairy-based treats), her weight loss resumed.

Too Few Calories

While it seems ridiculous at first glance, a major stumbling block is taking in too few calories. It is well accepted among seasoned reduced carbohydrate dieters and experts alike that a significant prolonged calorie deficit will cause the body to go into a state of seriously slowed metabolism, commonly referred to as "starvation mode."

Here is a fun way to think of this theory: Imagine a little weight control moderator who lives in your body. It is his job to ensure that your body has enough energy stored to get through lean times and periods of famine. He performs a valuable function, and without him, you could not survive. His job is to protect you. Now, imagine the moderator is seated before a big panel of monitors and other electronic devices with which he can keep a vigilant eye on all the events in your body. He can closely monitor events from here, and he can control your body's responses to them. The shortcoming is that this little fellow does not have a window from which he can view the world. He can only make judgments based upon the information he gets from the panel of monitors.

When you have an adequate calorie intake, the moderator is satisfied that plenty of fuel is coming into your body, and does not worry about the efficiency at which it is burned. He simply allows your body tissues to use whatever fuel they need, and, if any is left over, he stores it as fat in case your body needs it later. But if you restrict your calorie intake too much, he becomes vigilant about conserving energy. Remember, he does not have a window on the world. Although you know you have plenty of fuel available whenever you need it, he does not know that. He does not know if you are in the middle of the Sahara with no food in sight or in an overflowing grocery store.

So, when your calorie intake is too low, the moderator first releases some fat stores to make up for the deficit. However, he does not like to do this for a long period of time. Rather, he much prefers to conserve the stored fuel for a day when the situation is even worse. Therefore, instead of releasing large amounts of fat, he orders your body tissues to burn the available fuel more efficiently. If the fuel restriction is drastic, occurs suddenly, or lasts for a prolonged period, he will institute the emergency plan known as starvation mode. He will order your body to slow its processes so that less energy is required to keep you alive. In essence, he "turns down the heat" and "dims the lights."

For example, instead of needing 2,000 calories a day to function, your body will now need only 1,800 calories to keep things going. If this strategy is not fully successful and he still needs to use the fat stores more than he likes, he goes a step further. He begins to analyze which systems are less fuel-efficient than others. He quickly realizes that muscle requires much more energy to maintain than does fat, so he gives an order to dump muscle. He has now lowered your calorie requirements further. Besides, he knows the protein that is released when muscles are broken down can be converted to glucose and used as fuel. After he initiates these steps, he finds equilibrium between the incoming fuel and the body's need for it. The only problem is that the new equilibrium was struck at 1,600 calories per day—a level that is far below the original requirement of 2,000 calories per day.

Even after you resume taking in enough calories and the "emergency" is over, the moderator is likely to keep things running in this efficient mode for quite some time. For one reason, he is spooked. After the scare he experienced, he is not likely to trust that this renewed fuel source will last. At this point, he is very motivated to use any extra fuel coming in to replenish the fat stores that were lost. Second, your body has less muscle than it did before and requires less fuel function. The effect for you is that your rate of weight loss has slowed considerably.

While this starvation mode occurs on any diet plan that does not allow an adequate calorie intake, it can be especially troublesome on reduced carbohydrate diet plans for two reasons. First, after years of fighting hunger on low fat diets, new reduced carbohydrate dieters find that eating more protein and fat is much more satisfying than eating carbohydrate. These people may unintentionally restrict their calorie intake to inadequate levels because they are not accustomed to eating in the absence of overwhelming hunger and strong carbohydrate cravings; they simply forget to eat. This happened to Odele on several occasions. She reported to her fellow reduced carbohydrate dieters that she has experienced several episodes in which her appetite dipped to levels at which she was not motivated to eat.

The second factor relates to people on ketogenic diets. One of the treasured benefits of ketosis is that it can have a pronounced appetite-suppressing effect. Some people find themselves unable to resist the temptation of taking advantage of this loss of appetite in an attempt to drop large amounts of weight quickly. These people unwisely use appetite suppression as a tool to severely restrict their calorie intake.

Voice of Low Carb Experience

Seasoned low carbohydrate dieters rarely recommend that new reduced carbohydrate dieters count calories, since it is often counterproductive. Focusing on restricting calories in addition to counting carbohydrate grams can be quite an adjustment for people switching from a well-practiced low fat diet. However, you should be aware that there might be a time when you will need to consider calories. How do you know when that time has arrived? Your weight loss will slow significantly or stop altogether.

The key to success is to strike a balance between too many calories and too few calories. You should eat when you are hungry, but you should not eat until you are stuffed or overfilled; eat only until you are no longer hungry. On the other hand, you should not restrict your intake to the point of starving your body. If you find yourself without an appetite for a length of time, you must be careful not to take in significantly fewer calories than the range recommended for you or you will risk slow weight loss as a result of slowed metabolism.

Seasoned low carbohydrate dieters and some experts say that your daily calorie intake should be approximately 10 to 12 times your body weight. For example, if you weigh 200 pounds, your daily calorie intake should be between 2,000 and 2,400 calories. According to this guideline, as your body weight decreases, so should your calorie intake. The idea behind using a range of calories is to provide you with the flexibility to eat more calories on days when your hunger is greater and to eat less on days when your hunger is less. If you are a woman in your childbearing years, you already know that these hunger peaks and valleys can be especially pronounced at different points in your menstrual cycle. Using this approach, you should eat the higher number of calories on your "hungry" days and the lower number on normal days.

Protein

In the popular media, reduced carbohydrate eating plans are often labeled as high protein diets. Although some of us protest this, there is no debate among us that protein is a vital and necessary part of the reduced carbohydrate lifestyle. In fact, protein is widely believed to be the second most important key to achieving long-term success with dieting—second only to restricting carbohydrate. The rewards of eating adequate protein are many, not the least being increased satiety; protein keeps us satisfied longer.

But as with calories, you need to strike a balance between taking in too little protein and taking in too much. This is because protein is converted to blood glucose by our bodies through a process known as glucogenesis. (*Gluco* refers to the glucose, and *genesis* means "the creation of.") According to this theory, our bodies have the ability to create glucose from protein with an efficiency of about 50 percent. So if we consume too much protein, our bodies produce enough glucose to supply our energy needs without having to use our fat stores. One of the pieces of support for this theory is that some people who are on ketogenic diets find it hard to achieve or sustain ketosis even though they consistently keep their daily carbohydrate count low. For people who are not on ketogenic diets, the confirmation is that weight loss does not occur even though they keep their carbohydrate count down. In either case, the advocates of this theory believe that weight loss slows or stops in the presence of too much protein because the body no longer needs to dip into its fat stores to provide energy because it is provided through the process of glucogenesis.

Taking in too much protein can easily happen when we attempt to do a very low fat version of a low carbohydrate diet. By restricting carbohydrate *and* fat to low levels, we make up the bulk of our diet with protein. Not only does the excess protein slow our weight loss, overly restricting fat reduces our overall satiety and makes us more vulnerable to carbohydrate cravings.

At the same time, taking in too little protein has the same effect on our rate of weight loss as taking in too few calories. By failing to take in enough protein, we risk losing beneficial muscle mass. Reducing muscle slows our metabolism and either stalls our weight loss or stops it altogether. Taking in too little protein also sacrifices satiety, and our resulting hunger makes us much more vulnerable to carbohydrate cravings, a development that is definitely detrimental to our goal of reducing carbohydrate in our diet.

Voice of Low Carb Experience

The key to success is to take in enough protein to avoid muscle loss and to keep hunger in check, but not so much that you inflate your overall calorie count or stimulate excessive glucogenesis.

To determine how much protein you should consume daily, do a little research. The federal government's official recommended daily allowance for protein is 0.8 gram per kilogram of body weight per day, or, more generally, 50 grams per day for an "average" woman and 63 grams per day for an "average" man. A more individualized calculation explained in both *The Zone* and *Protein Power* is the most common approach used by reduced carbohydrate dieters. The authors of these books recommend consuming 0.5 to 0.9 gram of protein per pound of lean body mass, depending on your level of activity (ranging from 0.5 for sedentary persons up to 0.9 for athletes). For example, if a woman who weighs 167 pounds has a body fat percentage of 33 percent, she has approximately 55 pounds of fat (167 x 0.33 = 55). This means that she has approximately 112 pounds of lean body mass (167- 55 = 112). If she is mildly active, her minimum protein intake should be approximately 56 grams per day (112 x 0.5 = 56).

While this method allows you to tailor your protein intake according to your unique requirements, it requires that you know your lean body mass. To arrive at this estimate, you will need calipers or a body fat analyzer. These devices are available at most health clubs and medical offices or can be purchased at health-related stores. Both *The Zone* and *Protein Power* describe how to estimate lean body mass without using any devices. The method involves taking your body measurements and performing calculations in relation to your weight and height.

A quicker but less accurate method of estimating your minimum daily protein requirement is to multiply 0.5 gram of protein per pound of your total body weight. The shortcoming of this method is that the calculation is not based on the preferred indicator of lean body mass. Instead, it is based on total body weight, and people who have large amounts to lose are at risk for overestimating the amount of protein they can consume.

Regardless of the method you use to determine your minimum daily intake of protein, if you are experiencing very slow weight loss or a plateau, you should strive to balance your protein intake. First, be sure you are taking in enough protein according to the guidelines. Then, try to maintain your daily protein intake at a level that is only somewhat above the minimum recommended amount. For example, the woman used in the preceding example should first ensure that she is taking in at least 56 grams of protein per day. Then, she should adjust her protein intake so she is consuming an amount only slightly above the recommended 56 grams.

Increased Hunger

Many reduced carbohydrate dieters have noticed that a whoosh is often preceded by a period of increased hunger and strong carbohydrate cravings. While many women can correlate this to their menstrual cycle, men say they have also noticed this pattern. It is a common theory among seasoned reduced carbohydrate dieters that this is our bodies' last heroic effort to hold on to fat before letting it go.

Remember the moderator who regulates our bodies' metabolism? The moderator serves to protect us by balancing our energy needs with our available fuel by regulating our fat stores. For many people, the moderator does his job well and all is in balance. But for some of us, the moderator has a difficult time achieving equilibrium. He becomes anxious and overly worried that our fuel supply is going to run out, and he builds up our fat stores much more than necessary. He is obsessed and does not want to give up. He's like the rich man who has millions of dollars in the bank but walks around with holes in his shoes because he pinches his pennies simply for the sake of saving.

In the early days of a diet, when the moderator receives the signal to release some fat stores, he does so relatively easily. But a day arrives when the moderator notices your fat stores are getting much lower than they have been in a long time, maybe ever. He does not like it. He becomes nervous. He pulls out his bag of tricks. First, he simply refuses to release the fat. The incoming fuel is not enough to cover your body's needs, but he is stubborn, and he will not let go of the fat. Your weight loss slows or you hit a plateau. When the point arrives that the moderator must release some fat, he tries one last trick—his favorite. He sends up strong hunger pangs like emergency alarm bells. "That should do the trick," he thinks. "It always worked before."

Voice of Low Carb Experience

You can try having a conversation with your little moderator (although I highly recommend you do this in the privacy of your own home!) to let him know that you are on to his tricks and are not giving in. While this idea may bring a smile to your face and appear to be a bit of a joke, some dieters have found success by using self-hypnosis recordings, motivational meditations, or other methods of influencing their subconscious minds. Self-hypnosis recordings are commercially available at most bookstores, by mail order, and through web sites.

If you are not the sort who would enjoy the experience of self-hypnosis, there are other strategies available to manage increased hunger. First, look on this period as the dark before the dawn. If you stick with your plan during this dark period, you are much more likely to be rewarded with a whoosh when daylight arrives.

Second, while it is important to stick with the plan, it is also important not to deny yourself necessary food and allow your hunger to go unchecked. Now is the time to eat the higher levels of your recommended ranges of calories and protein. The best approach is to increase your intake of very low carbohydrate, high protein foods to satisfy your hunger. If your hunger is so great that even these higher levels do not satisfy it, eat until you are no longer hungry, even if it means going a bit over the recommended ranges. Remember, however, to eat only until you are no longer hungry, not until you are stuffed. Many reduced carbohydrate dieters keep plenty of low carbohydrate treats in ready-to-eat form on hand for emergencies. This practice can be a lifesaver when carbohydrate cravings are overwhelming.

Stubbornly refusing to eat more in the face of increased hunger can be counterproductive. You will be much more vulnerable to the carbohydrate siren song, and you may find that you are not able to resist it. This would be unfortunate because if you give in and eat too much carbohydrate, you risk having your weight loss slow or plateau (at best) or even gaining weight (at worst). And, since hunger is often worst immediately before a whoosh, you risk missing a whoosh!

Artificial Sweeteners

Among reduced carbohydrate dieters, there is a great deal of discussion about the pros and cons of artificial sweeteners in general and the role they play in slowing weight loss in particular. While some people use artificial sweeteners regularly and claim they have no real effect on their rate of weight loss, other people claim artificial sweeteners slow their weight loss to the point of causing stalls and plateaus.

Because there is such a wide divergence in opinions, discussions about artificial sweeteners are frequently lively. The topic is further muddled by a lack of agreement among the reduced carbohydrate diet book authors, some of whom advise eliminating all forms of artificial sweeteners, while others say it is acceptable to use them in limited quantities and still others say there is no need to be concerned at all. Furthermore, some of the reduced carbohydrate diet book authors have changed their opinions on the desirability of artificial sweeteners from one book to another, only adding to the confusion.

The most prevalent theory on how and why artificial sweeteners sabotage weight loss is that the mere taste of sweetness puts us into a nasty cycle of craving more sweet taste, which prompts us to overeat. While this theory is a major theme of the Hellers in *The Carbohydrate Addict's*

Diet, many of the other reduced carbohydrate diet book authors support it. These authors all believe that the taste of sweets, including artificial sweeteners, triggers the pancreas to release insulin *even when no carbohydrate is present.* The action of the insulin causes the blood glucose levels to fall, and the falling glucose levels cause hunger and carbohydrate cravings that lead us to overeat. Therefore, when we eat artificial sweeteners, the sweet taste triggers insulin releases that in turn slow our weight loss.

Randy has long suspected that he reacts to artificial sweeteners much the same way he reacts to sugar. He says that when he drinks a popular drink mix with artificial sweeteners in the hope of satisfying his sweet tooth, he is instead thrown into a cycle of craving more sweets. When he returns to drinking only water, his carbohydrate cravings go away.

Aspartame and Saccharin

The most frequently used artificial sweeteners in the United States are aspartame and saccharin. You know them well; they come in those familiar little pink or blue packets that adorn every restaurant table in the country. These sweeteners are used so often that reduced carbohydrate dieters often discuss a second theory on how artificial sweetners slow weight loss. According to this simple theory, we often overlook the fact that each of these little individual serving packets has approximately 1 gram of carbohydrate. If we use them frequently or in large amounts, we can unwittingly add significant amounts of carbohydrate to our daily totals. However, while this is a plausible explanation for many of us, there are others who say that even when they count the carbohydrate in them, their weight loss stalls.

Stevia

Because aspartame and saccharin have reputations for causing carbohydrate cravings and stalling weight loss, many reduced carbohydrate dieters use other artificial sweeteners. Stevia is a popular sweetener available at health food stores that many of us use successfully. Some people consider stevia a natural rather than an artificial sweetener because it is derived from the *Stevia rebaudiana* plant in a process similar to the one used to derive white sugar from sugarcane. Stevia has a much more concentrated sweet taste than artificial sweeteners do, and as a result, most people find they use very little of it, sometimes just a few drops per day. Stevia also has the added benefit of being available in a liquid form that has no carbohydrate.

However, stevia is not universally accepted by low carbohydrate dieters because many do not like the light licorice taste it sometimes has. The degree of its licorice taste is directly related to its degree of refinement; the more refined the product, the less it tastes like licorice. The least refined, most natural liquid version has a light to dark brown color and a moderate to strong licorice taste. The more refined liquid version is clear and has had much of its licorice taste removed in the processing. However, you should be aware that clear liquid stevia often contains glycerine, which can stall weight loss in and of itself. (For a discussion of glycerine, see pages 184–188.)

Stevia is also available in powdered form, with the degree of the licorice taste varying by brand. Some people say they notice the licorice taste only when they use a lot of stevia, so they combine the stevia with aspartame or saccharin. This dilutes the licorice taste. For example, Sally is a happy stevia user who says she much prefers it to aspartame and saccharin because of the carbohydrate savings. She discovered that most of her daily intake of artificial sweetener comes from the pitcher of decaffeinated tea she drinks each day. Instead of adding four packets of aspartame to each pitcher of tea, she now substitutes stevia for three of the packets without affecting the taste.

A word of caution: The FDA has declined repeatedly to approve stevia for use as an artificial sweetener. The FDA states there is insufficient data to prove its safety, although it has been used in Japan for more than 30 years without reports of harmful side effects. Since the FDA has little control over the marketing and sale of dietary supplements, stevia is therefore marketed and sold in the United States as a dietary supplement rather than an artificial sweetener.

Sucralose

A new artificial sweetener known as sucralose (distributed under the brand name of Splenda by Johnson & Johnson in the United States) has generated considerable excitement among low carbohydrate dieters, particularly among those who experience problems with aspartame and saccharin. Sucralose is sugar that has been modified into a form the body cannot digest. Because it is derived from real sugar, sucralose retains the taste of real sugar even when it is heated.

Although sucralose was used in Europe and Canada for several years, it was not approved by the FDA for general use in the United States until 1999. Therefore, it is just now making its way onto American supermarket shelves as an ingredient in products such as diet soft drinks and pancake syrup. It is also available in powdered and tablet form.

Sucralose itself has no carbohydrate, but the fillers that are added to it do. As a result, the powdered form contains approximately 1 gram of carbohydrate per packet, the same amount that aspartame and saccharin have. Even though powdered sucralose has the same carbohydrate count as aspartame and saccharin, it is not believed to slow weight loss. Although many people report using sucralose without any adverse affects, the question of whether or not it slows weight loss has yet to be fully answered.

Several low carbohydrate dieters who have tried sucralose have identified at least one shortcoming. They report that it tastes so much like table sugar that it triggers major carbohydrate cravings and precipitates significant carbohydrate binges for them. These people theorize that before using sucralose, they had become accustomed to living with the taste of artificial sweeteners or without the taste of sugar at all. In essence, they broke their carbohydrate addiction.

Richard believes that this is the case for him. He tells of his reaction after eating desserts he made with sucralose for a Thanksgiving dinner. Although he kept his carbohydrate count low, he said he had symptoms as though he had eaten real sugar. He gained weight and experienced the same carbohydrate hangover that many people describe after eating significant quantities of carbohydrate. Now, he says, he is much more hesitant to use sucralose except in small quantities.

Acesulfame-k

Acesulfame-k (sold under the brand name Sunette) is another recent addition to our arsenal of artificial sweeteners. Although it is new and does not lose its sweetness when heated, it has not received as much attention from low carbohydrate dieters as sucralose. Many people who try it say it is remarkably similar to aspartame in its taste and aftertaste, and this might explain why it has not produced the same amount of excitement as sucralose. Acesulfame-k is an ingredient in many sugar-free and low calorie products such as diet soft drinks, and it is also available in powdered form. As with all the other artificial sweeteners, each packet of the powdered form has about 1 gram of carbohydrate.

Voice of Low Carb Experience

To determine if artificial sweeteners slow your weight loss, stop using them for a trial period of two weeks. By the end of the two weeks, you should know whether they cause problems for you. If you are like many of us and cannot bear the thought of going without any sweet taste at all for two weeks, at least try to reduce the amount you use.

Fortunately for those of us who cannot live without some sweet taste in our diets, there are several methods that seasoned reduced carbohydrate dieters use to reduce the amount of artificial sweeteners they use. First, use stevia (if you like its taste), as it has a much more concentrated sweet taste and less of it is usually needed to achieve the desired sweetness in most foods. Another trick is to use small amounts of aspartame and saccharin together rather than using them individually. Many people report that mixing the two sweeteners increases their sugary taste and, therefore, they are able to use less. A third trick is to switch from powdered sweeteners to the liquid or tablet form. Most of the carbohydrate in powdered artificial sweeteners comes from the fillers, rather than from the sweetener itself. Most liquid sweeteners are carbohydrate-free, and the tablet forms have much lower carbohydrate counts. For example, the tablet form of aspartame has much less filler than does the powdered form; each tablet has only (0.1) gram of carbohydrate, as opposed to 1 gram of carbohydrate per packet of powder. Finally, sucralose is worth a try if you can afford it (it is fairly expensive at present).

Triggers

As already mentioned, one popular theory says that merely the taste of sweetness can slow weight loss. This theory is a major theme in *The Carbohydrate Addict's Diet*. According to the Hellers, the taste of sweetness is all that is necessary to activate a release of insulin. Actual carbohydrate need not be present. Like Pavlov's dogs, who reacted to the sound of a dinner bell by salivating even when food was not present, our pancreas reacts to the taste of sweetness by releasing insulin even when carbohydrate is not present. This insulin release causes our blood glucose levels to fall, and we develop symptoms related to low blood sugar as a consequence. Light-headedness, shakiness, sweating, fatigue, and nervousness are several symptoms frequently mentioned. The most significant symptoms, however, are hunger and carbohydrate cravings, particularly cravings for junk food and sweets. These cravings lead us to eat more than we need.

The foods and tastes that cause this reaction are commonly known as triggers because they trigger the insulin response that results in the carbohydrate cravings. Triggers can be foods, people, events, or situations that initiate an eating episode or pattern of eating that leads to weight gain. If we experience these triggers often enough, the resulting cycles can slow our weight loss.

This theory is well accepted among seasoned reduced carbohydrate dieters, although not everyone is affected. There are many stories told of carbohydrate binges that were set off by triggers. Sugar substitutes are notorious for triggering carbohydrate cravings. Other food triggers that are frequently mentioned are: products containing artificial sweeteners, caffeine, wine and other spirits, whipped cream, chocolate, nuts, and sugar-free snacks.

Voice of Low Carb Experience

Seasoned reduced carbohydrate dieters say that the best way to identify your personal triggers is to keep a food journal. Document all the food you eat along with when you eat it. Keep track of all strong carbohydrate cravings, increased hunger, or other symptoms of low blood sugar, as well as when they strike. If a food is your trigger, the most likely culprit will be something you ate about one to three hours before the craving struck. While this technique will not necessarily pinpoint all your carbohydrate triggers, it will help you narrow the possibilities. If you find the likely trigger is a food, omit it from your diet for at least two weeks to see if your cravings decrease.

If you are unable to identify a pattern; yet find yourself consistently challenged by strong carbohydrate cravings (especially if they are strong enough to cause you to overeat), omit all the triggers listed above one at a time for a couple of weeks to learn how they affect you.

And above all, if you find that something has triggered carbohydrate cravings and you are ambushed by the uncomfortable symptoms of low blood sugar, resist eating more sweets, whether they are made with real sugar or artificial sweeteners. Giving in and overeating carbohydrate will lead to a vicious cycle that eventually stalls your weight loss or, even worse, causes weight gain. Responding to the carbohydrate cravings by eating artificial sweeteners will only perpetuate the situation by triggering even stronger carbohydrate cravings later. Instead, eat a high protein, low carbohydrate food or a high fiber, low carbohydrate vegetable until you are satisfied. Protein, complex carbohydrate, and fiber raise blood glucose levels slowly without causing a further release of insulin, thereby breaking the destructive cycle.

Caffeine

Caffeine is a topic of frequent, lively discussions among reduced carbohydrate dieters, and it is one of the first offenders mentioned in any discussion about slow weight loss. Caffeine is the subject of considerable debate because the reduced carbohydrate diet book authors have conflicting views about it and their recommendations vary. Some of the authors recommend that caffeine be eliminated completely from the diet right at the beginning and not be reintroduced. They say caffeine stimulates the pancreas to release insulin even when the blood glucose levels are elevated. The insulin causes the blood glucose levels to drop, resulting in fatigue, irritability, hunger, and carbohydrate cravings. Other authors say caffeine should be eliminated in the early stages of the diet, but can be reintroduced later as long as you are not addicted to it. To further complicate the matter, other authors rigorously deny that caffeine causes any problems at all for reduced carbohydrate dieters and actually advocate using caffeine to *boost* weight loss. Still other authors say that caffeine is not a factor in either stalling or boosting weight loss.

The collective experience of the seasoned low carbohydrate dieters does little to clear the confusion. While some people find they are sensitive to caffeine and its removal results in major changes for them, others say that caffeine has no effect and they consume it at will.

Kimberly found that caffeine had a big impact on her rate of weight loss. During the first three months of her reduced carbohydrate diet, she refused to give up her beloved caffeine and found that her rate of weight loss was very slow. After she tried leaving out caffeine, she had positive results right away. She said that the week after her "hell week" of caffeine withdrawal was her best week of weight loss.

Voice of Low Carb Experience

If you consume caffeine, especially if you are addicted to it, you should consider eliminating it from your diet for several weeks to determine its effect on you. Remember, however, if you truly are addicted to caffeine, sudden withdrawal can cause a variety of unpleasant symptoms that can be a significant challenge. Headache, fatigue, and irritability are only three of the symptoms you may have if you quit cold turkey. Instead of suddenly removing caffeine, you may wish to choose a gradual approach, which seems to cause less discomfort. The idea is to reduce your intake in stages. For example, if you are accustomed to drinking three cups of coffee per day, reduce the amount to two cups for three days and then one cup for three days. You may get lucky and find along the way that your weight loss has accelerated and your body is doing better, so you don't have to eliminate caffeine completely.

Diet Soft Drinks

Among reduced carbohydrate dieters, diet soft drinks are widely believed to be one of the most common causes of slow weight loss. Diet soft drinks contain several ingredients that are believed to be culprits. They all have artificial sweeteners, most commonly aspartame, which slows weight loss in some people. Many also contain caffeine, another possible stumbling block. But even if you dodge both of these bullets and find that neither the artificial sweetener nor the caffeine slows your weight loss, another ingredient—citric acid—may be your downfall. Diet soft drinks can also be a source of unnecessary sodium, which often causes the body to retain water. This combination of artificial sweetener, caffeine, citric acid, and sodium makes diet soft drinks a potential weight loss disaster in one small package.

Voice of Low Carb Experience

Diet soft drinks should be the first thing to go when your weight loss slows or you find yourself stuck in a plateau. The idea is that you get a lot of bang for your buck here. Eliminating diet soft drinks removes four of the biggest diet hazards—artificial sweeteners, caffeine, citric acid, and sodium—in one fell swoop. If you are unlucky and are sensitive to all these ingredients, this one action alone could make a huge difference in your rate of weight loss.

Glycerine

Glycerine is a food additive frequently used in sugar-free products to provide sweetness and texture as a sugar substitute. In fact, glycerine is so common that most low carbohydrate snack products, including those popular high protein snack bars, list it as one of their first ingredients. While the mere presence of glycerine is not a point of serious controversy, how the glycerine is counted on the Nutrition Facts label is. Here is the central question: Should glycerine be counted as a carbohydrate or not? Some food producers say no because in most people, glycerine is not metabolized as a carbohydrate and, therefore, does not raise the blood sugar levels. However, many dieters dispute this point and claim that in some people, glycerine is metabolized very much like carbohydrate and, therefore, raises the blood sugar levels. They argue that glycerine should be included in the total carbohydrate count.

To add to the controversy, many food producers have an unusual practice of including glycerine in the total calorie count while excluding it from the carbohydrate, protein, and fat counts. This practice is controversial because carbohydrate, protein, and fat are the only three macronutrients our bodies use as sources of nutrition. Therefore, if a substance contributes calories to the diet, it should also be included in either the carbohydrate, protein, or fat count. Omitting glycerine from the carbohydrate, protein, and fat counts while including it in the total calorie count creates an "unbalanced" Nutrition Facts label.

To illustrate this point, Figure 3.5 shows the Nutrition Facts label and ingredient list from a low carbohydrate, high protein snack bar that I bought at my local health food store. Glycerine is the second ingredient on the ingredient list, but it is not included in the total carbohydrate count, which is given as a very low 2.6 grams per bar. However, the manufacturer does acknowledge the glycerine controversy on the label. Two asterisks (**) included with the total carbohydrate count correspond to the following statement: "Glycerine and polydextrose, while included in the calorie count, have been omitted from the 'Total Carb' count, as they have only a negligible impact on blood sugar levels."

To confirm this statement, I quickly reviewed the label. It lists the total fat content as 13 grams per bar, which works out to 117 calories, since fat contains 9 calories per gram. The protein content is listed as 18 grams per serving, which is 72 calories, since protein has 4 calories per gram. The carbohydrate count is given as 2.6 grams, which, since carbohydrate has 4 calories per gram, works

Nutrition Facts
Serving Size 1 bar (60g)

Amount Per Serving	
Calories 240	**Calories from Fat** 117

	% Daily Value*
Total Fat 13g	**20%**
Saturated Fat 7g	**35%**
Cholesterol 5mg	**2%**
Sodium 196mg	**8%**
Total Carbohydrate 2.6g **	**1%**
Fiber 1g	**4%**
Sugars 0g	**0%**
Protein 18g	**36 %**

*Percent Daily Values are based on a 2,000 calorie diet.

INGREDIENTS: Isolated soy protein, glycerine, polydextrose, water, whey protein isolate, natural palm kernel oil, lecithin, calcium, sodium caseinate, ghee (clarified butter), natural coconut oil, high oleic sunflower oil, macadamia nuts, cocoa, natural flavors, potassium chloride, citric acid, sucralose, potassium sorbate. *(Author's Note: The label also contained several vitamins that are not listed here.)*

Figure 3.5. Even though glycerine is the second item in this ingredient list, it is omitted from the total carbohydrate count, creating an unbalanced Nutrition Facts label.

out to approximately 10 calories. The calories from fat, protein, and carbohydrate add up to only 199 calories per bar, however, while the total is listed as 240 calories. This is a difference of 41 calories. According to the statement on the label, the difference between the calories we calculated and the total calories given on the label is due to the glycerine it contains.

Reduced carbohydrate dieters who are sensitive to glycerine would use this calorie difference as the basis for estimating a revised carbohydrate count. By dividing the missing 41 calories by 4 (the number of calories attributed to the glycerine divided by the number of calories per gram of carbohydrate), they would estimate that the glycerine could have a metabolic effect similar to that of 10.25 grams of carbohydrate for those who are sensitive to it.

Occasionally, people on ketogenic diets find that eating glycerine-based snacks causes their ketosis to immediately diminish or disappear for several hours. They consider this to be clear evidence that their bodies are indeed metabolizing glycerine as carbohydrate. Other dieters, including many not on ketogenic diets, report that eating glycerine-based snacks stalled their weight loss.

On the other hand, many reduced carbohydrate dieters report they are able to consume glycerine daily without any noticeable problems. These people love glycerine-based snacks and often use them as meal replacements if they are otherwise unable to get low carbohydrate food. For example, Jean travels a great deal for her job and finds eating in airports extremely difficult. She says that she never goes on a trip without several low carbohydrate snack bars in her bag. She says that having them readily available has saved her from falling victim to high carbohydrate airport food during long layovers and lengthy flight delays.

Voice of Low Carb Experience

As is the case with most controversies, the best way to handle glycerine in your diet is a compromise of what the two opposing sides recommend. Because this possible stumbling block is highly individualized, you must do your own experiments to find out if it is a problem for you. If you are in ketosis, consider testing your urine for the presence of ketones and then eating a low carbohydrate snack bar that contains glycerine. Retesting your urine two to three hours later may let you know immediately if glycerine has an effect on you. Even if you do not notice an immediate effect on your ketosis, or if you are not on a ketogenic diet, you should eliminate glycerine for a trial period of at least two weeks.

If you find you are sensitive to glycerine, choose snacks that do not contain it. In response to the controversy, several manufacturers of low carbohydrate snacks are developing products that are glycerine-free. Several of these products are available now, and more are on the way.

On the other hand, if you are not sensitive to glycerine, you should not worry about avoiding the snacks that contain it. They can be great emergency meal replacements when no alternatives are available.

Alcohol

Some of the most common questions new reduced carbohydrate dieters ask of seasoned dieters relate to the effects of alcohol. Few other topics draw so many conflicting responses. For this debate, the field is wide open for interpretation, as there is no clear agreement among the seasoned dieters or the experts on whether alcohol hinders weight loss or not.

Essentially, there are two schools of thought on this issue. One school believes that alcohol definitely inhibits weight loss and induces stalls. These dieters give anecdotal evidence of long plateaus that were broken only after they gave up alcohol. Their theory is that our bodies use alcohol as fuel before body fat, thereby slowing weight loss. The other school argues that alcohol can actually benefit reduced carbohydrate dieters by increasing our ability to use insulin effectively. Looking to the reduced carbohydrate diet books to reconcile these two opposing views provides little help because the authors also directly disagree with one another.

Perhaps the most persuasive case for restricting or eliminating alcohol is that it can seriously weaken our resistance to high carbohydrate temptations. Many mournful confessions are made the day following parties and festivities by people who painfully regret making the mistake of drinking alcohol in the presence of the abundance of high carbohydrate goodies that lurk at every celebration.

For example, Amelia attempted to isolate the cause of her overwhelming evening carbohydrate cravings for more than five months. She was puzzled because during the day, she was not tempted by sweets in the least, but after dinner, she had strong cravings and would find herself in her kitchen searching for sugar. She found that these strong urges caused her to overeat carbohydrate to the point that her weight loss stalled. But even worse, the cravings and her resulting plateau upset and discouraged her so much that she felt like a failure, especially when she compared herself to her reduced carbohydrate dieting peers. During the five months in which she tried to isolate her triggers, she omitted artificial sweeteners, diet soft drinks, and low carbohydrate treats, but evening cravings continued to plague her. Then for two weeks, she left out the glass of dry white wine that she drank each evening with dinner. She saw immediate results: Her evening cravings completely disappeared. Later, as an experiment, she added the wine back to her dinner, and she once again found herself with her hand "deep, deep, deep in the cookie jar." She says she is greatly relieved to know her evening cravings are now under control.

Voice of Low Carb Experience

As for all potential stumbling blocks, the best advice is to eliminate alcohol for a couple of weeks to see if it has been slowing your weight loss or triggering carbohydrate cravings. If alcohol does seem to cause problems for you, eliminate it. If you find alcohol does not hinder your weight loss and choose to resume drinking it, consider doing so infrequently and lightly. If you prefer to drink wine, choose one that is dry rather than sweet; this will save you several grams of carbohydrate. If you prefer to drink hard liquor or other spirits, be cautious of the carbohydrate in the mixers.

Medications and Nutritional Supplements

The list of medications and nutritional supplements that have the potential to undermine weight loss on reduced carbohydrate diets is long enough to be the topic of a separate book. In the interest of brevity, let us just say here that many reduced carbohydrate dieters who were once losing weight very slowly report that their rate of weight loss accelerated after discontinuing medications or nutritional supplements.

Voice of Low Carb Success

You should never discontinue a medication without first consulting with your physician, especially if it was prescribed to treat a medical condition or illness. However, some people find that as their weight falls, their overall health improves, the underlying illness gets better, and they need less medication. For example, hypertension is closely linked with obesity, and many people find that as their weight drops, their blood pressure also drops and they need less medication to treat it. If you think this may be the case for you, consult your physician about the necessity of continuing your medications in light of your improved medical condition. You may find that you are one of the lucky ones who can safely give up prescription medication after years of taking it.

If you find that you must continue to take your prescription medication, consult with your pharmacist and the drug company to determine if the medication contains significant amounts of carbohydrate. If so, your pharmacist may be able to recommend a sugar-free or carbohydrate-free alternative. The Stanford University School of Medicine Department of Pediatrics maintains a web site that contains a review of the carbohydrate content of several prescription medications. While the site does not provide actual carbohydrate counts for the given medications, it does state whether or not the medications contain carbohydrate. The web site address is http://www.stanford.edu/group/ketodiet.

In addition to reviewing your prescription medications, you and your physician should also review all the over-the-counter medications and nutritional supplements you are taking to ensure they are necessary. You should eliminate the unnecessary ones for at least two weeks to determine their effects on your rate of weight loss. You should try to find out if the ones you and your physician feel are necessary contain any carbohydrate. Most people are surprised to learn that one of the most deeply hidden sources of carbohydrate is the "filler" added to medications, vitamins, and nutritional supplements (including fiber preparations such as psyllium husks). For example, Marilee was very surprised to find dextrose (a sugar) in the chewable antacid she used regularly.

If the item is an over-the-counter medication or dietary supplement, you should be able to determine if it contains carbohydrate by reading the ingredient list on the package. Sources of hidden carbohydrate are most often listed in the inactive ingredient list, rather than in the active ingredient list, but they can appear in either one. Many over-the-counter medications, including cough syrups and throat lozenges, are available in sugar-free forms and can be found in the diabetic sections of pharmacies. If you cannot locate a diabetic version on the shelf, you may be able to special order one through your pharmacy. There are also several Internet web sites that specialize in low sugar, sugar-free, and carbohydrate-free medications and supplements. While some of the low sugar and sugar-free medications may have some carbohydrate in them, they will contain less carbohydrate than their sugar-laden counterparts.

A word of caution: In your quest to discontinue all unnecessary medications and dietary supplements, you should not discontinue taking a high-quality multivitamin. The benefits of taking a multivitamin are many, whether or not you are dieting. When it comes to weight loss, it can help reduce food cravings caused by vitamin deficiencies.

Underactive Thyroid

For some of us, the cause of our slow weight loss may be an internal problem rather than an external one. It is well known in the medical community that the thyroid gland plays an important role in regulating the metabolism. Hypothyroidism, the name for the condition in which the thyroid is underactive, is characterized by a slowing of body functions. Because a sluggish thyroid drags down the metabolism, people with an underactive thyroid struggle with slow weight loss, plateaus, and chronic weight gain.

Hypothyroidism is a fairly common condition, affecting approximately 1 to 2 percent of the U.S. population. It is believed to be commonly underdiagnosed, especially in women and in people who are over 60 years old. The onset of the illness tends to be gradual, and the symptoms may go unrecognized until the condition worsens. The symptoms reflect the general slowing of the body's functions and include fatigue, lethargy, sleepiness, depression, weight gain, mental impairment, decreased appetite, cold intolerance, decreased perspiration, hoarseness, dry skin, dry and brittle hair, brittle nails, hair loss, generalized swelling and water retention, slow wound healing, constipation, menstrual irregularities, and infertility.

Diagnosing hypothyroidism is relatively simple because several blood tests are available that readily measure the levels of the thyroid hormones in the body. However, there is some controversy in the medical community about whether the standard tests reveal all cases of hypothyroidism. For some people, more extensive testing may be required. Treatment also is relatively simple, since there are several thyroid hormone drugs, some synthetic and some natural, that replace the body's missing thyroid hormones.

For example, Jewel's hypothyroidism was undiagnosed for years, although she was actively treated for depression and her weight steadily climbed. When she was finally diagnosed, she was placed on thyroid hormone replacement therapy, and she found she was finally able to lose weight.

Voice of Low Carb Experience

If you are experiencing very slow weight loss and the symptoms of hypothyroidism, you should consider that you may have an underactive thyroid. An easy home test is to take your temperature with a glass thermometer before you get out of bed each morning for a week. Women who have menstrual cycles should begin on the second or third day of their period (preferably the second day), since menstrual cycles affect body temperature. If your oral temperature is consistently below 97.8° to 98.0°F, and if you experience at least some of the symptoms of an underactive thyroid, you should consult your physician.

Yeast Overgrowth

Although yeast overgrowth is not frequently discussed among reduced carbohydrate dieters, some of the diet experts list it as a potential cause of slow weight loss and plateaus. Yeast overgrowth is a syndrome in which *Candida albicans,* a common yeast present in all our bodies, begins to overgrow, causing a variety of unpleasant symptoms and problems including weight gain and slow weight loss. Yeast overgrowth has been researched and publicized in several books, the most popular of which is *The Yeast Connection* by Dr. William G. Crook (Vintage Books, 1986).

The proponents of this theory say that the primary cause of yeast overgrowth is the overuse of antibiotics. The idea is that our bodies house several varieties of bacteria that are beneficial to our health. Normally, these bacteria keep the yeast in our bodies in check and prevent it from overgrowing. However, when we take antibiotics, we kill these beneficial bacteria along with the offending bacteria and the yeast begins to grow unchecked.

Another reason often cited for yeast overgrowth is the large amount of sugar in our diets. Yeast thrives on sugar, and since our sugar intake has dramatically increased over the past several years, so have the organisms that feed on it. Other causes often cited for yeast overgrowth are pregnancy (especially multiple pregnancies), birth control pills, steroids, and exposure to a variety of chemicals.

Vaginal yeast infection is the most common result of yeast overgrowth. However, yeast can also overgrow in the bowel and other important organs, in both men and women. The symptoms of yeast overgrowth are somewhat generalized and often difficult to pin down. They are believed to be caused by the toxins that the yeast produces. For example, the most common complaint is a chronic feeling of fatigue and lethargy. Other major symptoms are drowsiness, depression, numbness, burning, tingling, muscle aches, muscle weakness, joint pain, abdominal pain, constipation or diarrhea, bloating, belching, intestinal gas, vaginal burning and itching with a discharge, prostatitis, impotence, loss of sexual desire, endometriosis, infertility, cramps and other menstrual irregularities, premenstrual tension, anxiety attacks or crying, low body temperature with cold hands and feet, hypothyroidism, shaking and irritability when hungry, and bladder irritation.

Two low carbohydrate diet experts, Dr. Atkins and Dr. Pescatore, strongly believe that yeast overgrowth is a major cause of slow weight loss and plateaus, and they devote significant portions of their books to the topic. However, other reduced carbohydrate experts discount yeast overgrowth as a valid syndrome, and they have plenty of company. The yeast overgrowth theory has received sharp criticism from the medical community, primarily because of the lack of acceptance of an objective medical test that proves the existence of yeast overgrowth coupled with the generalized nature of the symptoms. Some reduced carbohydrate dieters report that when they sought advice from their physicians about yeast overgrowth, they were not taken seriously and their physician refused to consider it a potential problem for them. One of the recommended methods for diagnosing the syndrome is to take prescription medications known to kill yeast to see if the symptoms clear. However, this can be difficult, since physicians generally are unwilling to prescribe trial runs of the medications.

Several yeast and herbal experts provide detailed information in their books about herbal preparations and other supplements reputed to kill yeast. These remedies include *Lactobacillus acidophilus, Lactobacillus plantarum, Lactobacillus bulgaricus, Lactobacillus casei,* pau d'arco, garlic, *Bifido bacterium,* caprylic acid, undecenylic acid, tanalbit, olive leaf extract, oil of oregano, citrus seed extract, ozone, hydrogen peroxide, chlorine dioxide, and chlorophyll concentrate.

A word of caution: Before you take any of these over-the-counter preparations, you should thoroughly research and discuss with your physician the potential benefits and risks associated with them.

Voice of Low Carb Experience

While yeast overgrowth is not one of the more frequently discussed reasons for slow weight loss, you may wish to consider it as a possibility if all your other attempts to speed your weight loss or break a plateau fail. Research the syndrome thoroughly to see if the symptoms apply. Several books and web sites are devoted to the topic, and many of them have questionnaires for self-evaluation. After you have done the research and concluded that yeast overgrowth might be a problem, you should discuss it with your physician. Treatment of yeast overgrowth can be somewhat complex, and the guidance of a knowledgeable physician is extremely beneficial.

Some dietary changes may be of benefit if you believe yeast may be a problem. While a reduced carbohydrate diet naturally reduces the sugar and yeasted breads that aggravate the problem, you may also find it necessary to restrict other fermented and yeast-containing foods such as cheese, vinegar, mushrooms, wine, and beer.

Sodium

One of the great aspects of reduced carbohydrate dieting for many of us is that we do not retain as much water as we did in our high carbohydrate diet days. It is widely known that carbohydrate in our diets leads to water retention in our bodies. Therefore, if we eat less carbohydrate, we hold less water. Medically, this release of water is known as diuresis. Diuresis is especially marked for people who are on very low carbohydrate or ketogenic diets.

Diuresis is widely viewed as a great benefit of low carbohydrate dieting, as many people who had problems with water retention in the past find they are no longer struggling with it. Often, these folks are delighted to find they no longer need to limit their sodium intake to control water retention as long as they limit their carbohydrate intake.

However, after a while on a low carbohydrate diet (usually several months), some people report that their bodies adjust and consuming too much salt can once again trigger water retention. This return of water retention is pesky in that it not only makes people physically uncomfortable, but it can also mask their fat loss.

Jocelyn found this out the hard way. She loved it when she discovered early in her low carbohydrate diet that she no longer had to restrict her salt intake. But after a while, she began to notice that eating salty foods was once again causing her to retain some water, which would show as a slight gain on the scale the next morning. For example, after eating a sausage and sauerkraut dish and drinking a diet soft drink for dinner one evening, she woke the next morning to find she had gained 5 pounds. While she knew that a weight gain of that magnitude in such a short period of time was temporary, she was saddened to realize she would once again have to monitor her salt intake.

People who are troubled by water retention are often advised to restrict their sodium intake because sodium causes our bodies to hold water, and most of us get too much of it. We only need about 1,000 to 2,000 milligrams of sodium per day. A single teaspoon of table salt already contains 2,000 milligrams of sodium, and sodium is a component of many other foods. Nearly any ingredient listed on a product package that contains the term "sodium," such as monosodium glutamate or sodium nitrate, contains sodium. When we include a lot of foods like this in our daily sodium count, many of us find that we take in much more sodium than we need.

While it seems counterproductive at first, the best way to rid our bodies of retained water is to drink more water. Drinking more water flushes excess sodium from our bodies, and without the extra sodium, our bodies will not hold as much fluid. A fun, simple way to think about the relationship between sodium and water is to imagine that sodium and water are on the opposite ends of the rope in a tug-of-war game. The rope is never slack; there is constant tension between the end that is controlled by the sodium and the end that is controlled by the water. The body is constantly trying to keep these two opposing forces in balance because both sodium and water are necessary for it to function properly. Ideally, neither side is winning and neither side is losing. The little flag that marks the middle of the rope is exactly in the middle. The body is not dehydrated, nor is it bloated with excess fluid. It is in balance.

But then something happens. The person who lives in the body eats a bag of salty pork rinds and drinks a diet soft drink. Pork rinds contain approximately 1,500 milligrams of sodium, and diet soft drinks contain approximately 50 milligrams. Suddenly, sodium begins to win the tug-of-war. The body is now out of balance. Too much sodium is present, and not enough water is there to offset it.

The body first quickly checks to see if any water is coming along with the sodium, but, in this example, the owner of the body did not drink water with the pork rinds; he drank a diet soft drink instead. The body determines that there does not appear to be any hope of getting any extra water soon and that it must make do with what it has. Therefore, it sends an emergency signal to the kidneys to stop releasing water and to recycle it to provide reinforcements to the water end of the rope. The kidneys respond, and the release of water is stopped. All the water that is available to the body is held to offset the sodium's strength. The extra water is put in place to recover balance and the center of the rope returns to its original position.

However, things are not as they were before. While the body was able to restore balance and the flag is back in the middle, much more sodium is now present and much more water is on both sides of the rope. The extra sodium is not allowing the extra water to be released, and body tissues are beginning to swell. The swelling is uncomfortable, but the body is stubborn and is not going to let go of any extra water until the sodium loses its strength. If more water does not arrive, the body will continue to hold the water to remain at its new point of equilibrium.

The person who lives in the body steps on the scale the next morning and learns that he gained 3 pounds overnight. But he is smart and understands the relationship between sodium and water, and he begins the day by drinking a large bottle of water. Suddenly, everything shifts again. The water end of the rope is now much stronger than the sodium end. The water end is so strong that it defeats the sodium end. In fact, the body quickly gives the kidneys the signal that all is well and the kidneys release water once again. As the water is released, the extra sodium is washed away with the excess water. Once again, the body's sodium and water are in balance at a much lower, and much more comfortable, water level.

Voice of Low Carb Experience

If you are experiencing slow weight loss or are stuck in a stall, you should reduce your sodium intake and increase your water intake for a couple of weeks to see if water retention may be masking your fat loss. Even if water retention was not a problem early in your diet, your body may be adjusting and you may be retaining excess water now. For immediate feedback, increase the amount of water you drink right away. Many people find that by decreasing their sodium intake at the same time they increase their water intake, they can see results in 24 to 48 hours. As is discussed more fully in Chapter 4, those of us with normal kidney function should drink at least 64 ounces of water per day, plus an additional 8 ounces for each 25 pounds of weight we need to lose.

Monosodium Glutamate

Many reduced carbohydrate dieters, particularly those who follow the Carbohydrate Addict's Diet, believe that monosodium glutamate, commonly known as MSG, slows weight loss and contributes to stalls and plateaus. MSG is a food additive used to enhance the taste of foods and is frequently found in snack foods, processed meats, and oriental dishes. Some dieters report that MSG triggers carbohydrate cravings and lowers their resistance to carbohydrate temptations.

Abbey learned this disturbing lesson during her vacation. While at a world-famous resort, she ate Chinese food, a cuisine she had rarely eaten since beginning her low carbohydrate diet more than a year before. Despite the fact that the meal was very low carbohydrate, in about two hours she had the strongest carbohydrate cravings and hunger that she had experienced in the past year. She struggled with these strong cravings for nearly two days. Although Abbey could not be absolutely certain that MSG was the culprit, she now avoids MSG diligently.

Voice of Low Carb Experience

While MSG is not frequently mentioned by reduced carbohydrate dieters as a factor that slows weight loss, it does seem to affect some people. You may wish to steer clear of foods containing MSG for a week or two to see if it has an impact on the degree of your carbohydrate cravings and the speed of your weight loss.

Psychological Limitations

While it may be difficult to face, some people have found that their primary stumbling block is an emotional rather than a physical one. Many experienced dieters have come to accept that there are really two types of hunger. The type that generates the most open discussion is the physical need for food as a source of nutrition. The second type is a psychological craving for food as a source of emotional comfort. This latter type of hunger is not as freely discussed in casual conversations, but it is discussed more openly in weight loss support groups.

It is difficult work to decipher the reasons we use food (and the resulting extra weight) as psychological comfort. Many people find that as they lose weight, the psychological comfort the extra weight brought is removed, making them uncomfortable. The consensus among seasoned dieters is that outside attention to lost weight begins to snowball at around 35 pounds. They found that, for some reason, friends and coworkers began to comment regularly at this point about their weight loss. When the attention arrives, so does the psychological discomfort for many people, and this discomfort may result in self-defeating behavior that can slow or stop weight loss.

One reason the mind can be a stumbling block is that losing significant amounts of weight can alter our relationships with our friends, family, and the rest of the world, and we may not be emotionally ready. This can be especially true if you lose a great deal of weight or lose it very quickly. The sudden change in how you are treated can be unsettling, and you may unintentionally slow things down to regain some of the psychological comfort that melted away with the extra weight.

For example, Margarite found that after losing 98 pounds on a low carbohydrate plan, her weight loss stopped. At first, she thought her body needed a period of adjustment, but later, she discovered it was really her spirit that needed the adjustment period. She knew what it was like to be overlooked and ignored by people because of her weight. She thought she resented it, and she complained about it regularly. But some time during her very long plateau, she realized (with the help of her best friend) that she really had the opposite problem. As she was nearing an average size, she began to get some unexpected and unwanted attention from men. One day, as she and her best friend were shopping, a man approached her and flirted without invitation. Her friend noticed her body language during the encounter and commented that the flirting appeared to disturb Margarite. Margarite said the comment struck her like a bolt of lightning. She realized she was being forced to deal with an issue that had long been buried: her deep-seated resentment that she was judged by her body size. It angered her that men who would not have given her the time of day in the past now seemed hungry for her attention. Was she not the same person she was 98 pounds ago? She slowly came to realize that the layers of weight she had carried gave her some protection from the world. When she was larger, she knew that those people who were her friends, including her husband, valued her because of her personality and character, not because of her appearance. When her weight became low enough that she reentered male radars, she lost a little of the psychological "stealth" protection her weight had given her, and it made her uncomfortable. Her weight loss stopped. Margarite realized her extra weight was a form of insulation from the world. As she peeled the insulation away, she felt vulnerable, and her weight loss stalled. Once she realized her plateau was really caused by her discomfort with losing her social anonymity, she was able to deal with it and move forward.

Gayle agrees with Margarite that it is disturbing to be evaluated according to body size. She says she encountered a roadblock when she realized she had mental resistance to becoming one of the people she had disliked for much of her life, starting as far back as grade school. She realized that over the years, she had developed a subconscious belief that people who were overweight were more enlightened than their thinner counterparts. She believed that being overweight heightened her ability to judge people by their inner beauty rather than their physical appearance. She worried that once she became thin, she would lose her sensitivity for others and would join those who she believed valued physical appearance too much.

Some seasoned reduced carbohydrate dieters believe that a psychological stall is our psyche's quiet message that we need time to emotionally adjust to our weight loss before we can move forward. Helen describes this psychological adjustment as allowing her "sense of size to catch up with her." She says that after she loses a substantial amount of weight, she begins to feel very skinny. When this skinny feeling begins to disturb her, she backs off a bit and goes on a maintenance diet to maintain the new low weight. She says she knows when her psyche is ready to resume losing weight because it gives her a signal: She begins to feel heavy again. She finds this curious because her size and scale weight are the same as they were when she felt skinny and uncomfortable.

Voice of Low Carb Experience

If your weight loss is very slow, or if you have been stuck in a long plateau, you should consider the psychological impact losing weight may be having on you, especially if you have lost a great deal of weight or lost it very quickly. You need to be kind to yourself and realize that if you spent a long time, maybe even most of your life, as an overweight person, your weight loss may be having a significant impact on your emotional security, as well as on your relationships with your family, friends, and outside world.

Many seasoned reduced carbohydrate dieters have experienced psychological stumbling blocks and triumphed over them. They say the first step is to recognize that this internal confusion exists and is blocking your ability to lose more weight. Recognizing it as a barrier to your weight loss is a good sign that you are psychologically ready to deal with it. Take stock and reevaluate why you wanted to lose weight in the first place. Once your goals and dreams are firmly replanted in your head, they can motivate you to get back on track. But that is not enough. You must recognize that there is a bit of a battle going on between your head and your heart. Simply reminding yourself of the cognitive reasons you want to lose weight will not motivate your psyche to move forward. So, in addition to reminding yourself of why you wish to be thin, you must also identify the comfort the extra weight brings you. We all have reasons we are comfortable with our extra weight. Try to be honest with yourself about why you may be subconsciously holding on to the extra pounds. Writing a pro and con list can be a big help because, although they are very dear to us, our reasons for being overweight are never really very good. Bringing them to the surface and taking the time to deal with them often lessens their power over us.

If this is the case for you, listen to your psyche's quiet message and take the time to do the psychological work that will allow you to move forward. By sorting out the emotional impact your weight loss is having on you and others, you will be much more likely to sustain your weight loss, rather than regain the weight in a subconscious attempt to return your relationships back to "normal." This process may take some time. It cannot be rushed. You should trust your instincts; you will know when you are comfortable enough to proceed again. A word of caution: While you are working out the reasons for your psychological plateau, you should continue your diet. Many people eat just enough carbohydrate to cause their weight loss to stop, but not enough to gain any weight back until they are psychologically ready to lose more weight.

(For more information on the psychology of dieting, see *The Carbohydrate Addict's Diet* and *Thin for Good.*)

Fatigue

For many of us, lack of sleep has an effect similar to that of alcohol: It weakens our ability to resist carbohydrate and lures us to overeat. This connection is so strong for some people that they can directly correlate the degree of their fatigue to the degree of their overeating. Why fatigue leads to overeating is not completely clear, but many peo-

ple say it is as though their bodies confuse the fatigue that
results from lack of sleep with the fatigue that occurs with
low blood sugar. As a result, these people mistakenly believe their bodies are telling them that if they eat, especially carbohydrate, their energy will return.

While this can happen to anyone, for those people whose
extra weight causes sleep disorders such as serious snoring
and sleep apnea (a condition in which snoring is so severe
that the airway is temporarily blocked and the person is
unable to breathe for a short period), this can be a chronic,
vicious cycle. Serious snoring and sleep apnea are often associated with overweight, particularly when the extra fat is
stored in the upper body, neck, and face. Because serious
snoring and sleep apnea disturb normal sleep patterns, a
chronic state of fatigue results that, in turn, causes a
chronic state of carbohydrate cravings. Sufferers find
themselves in a downward spiral in that the more they
overeat, the heavier they get, the worse their sleep disorder becomes, and the poorer the quality of the sleep they
get. It becomes a destructive, self-enforcing cycle that
leads to chronic weight gain.

Robert is a prime example of this pattern. Like many
men, he carried the bulk of his extra weight in his upper
body, around his waist, chest, and neck. This extra weight
led him to develop sleep apnea in his fifties. His sleep
apnea became so serious that he was chronically fatigued.
He says it seemed the more fatigued he was, the hungrier
he was. Becoming motivated to exercise was clearly out of
the question. All he wanted to do was eat and sleep.

Robert was unable to break this destructive cycle until
he sought medical intervention for his sleep apnea. After
his treatment, he began to get quality sleep on a regular
basis, his energy returned, and his resistance to carbohydrate improved. He began to lose weight. In the first year

of low carbohydrate eating (and walking regularly), he lost 75 pounds.

The cause of fatigue need not be as dramatic as in Robert's case. Elizabeth agrees that fatigue definitely contributes to her weight loss stalls. She works in a profession prone to sudden increases in workload to meet client deadlines. She says she noticed that when her job is chaotic and she is working many extra hours, her carbohydrate cravings increase, her ability to resist them decreases, and her weight loss slows. Once her schedule returns to normal and she is able to catch up on sleep, her weight loss resumes.

Voice of Low Carb Experience

Many people report that their sleep disturbances such as snoring and sleep apnea improved as their weight decreased (much to their spouses' delight!). For these people, losing weight broke the fatigue/weight-gain cycle. However, other people find that medical intervention is necessary to get out of this destructive cycle. If your family tells you that you have serious snoring or sleep apnea, you should consult a physician. If you are not sure you have one of these sleep disturbances, or you are certain that you do not but are chronically fatigued, consulting your physician might still help you to sort out all the causes of your fatigue.

If you experience short-term sleep deprivation, such as when a new baby arrives, recognize that you may experience increased carbohydrate cravings in a subconscious effort to increase your energy level. Keep a lot of legal foods and treats in reach to combat these cravings and make getting plenty of sleep a priority.

Smoking

The evils of smoking have been cited by the United States Surgeon General's office for years. Now you can add a couple more negative effects to the list. Several reduced carbohydrate diet experts believe that smoking has a pronounced negative effect on the body's ability to properly metabolize carbohydrate. They cite medical research that confirms that smoking contributes to the development of insulin resistance and type II diabetes.

Voice of Low Carb Experience

If you smoke, quit. Do it soon. The most common reason people give for not quitting while dieting is the fear that their weight will rebound. However, several people who successfully quit smoking while dieting report that they found it easier to quit while on a reduced carbohydrate diet than at any other time.

If you think any of the factors discussed in this chapter may be a problem for you, take the time necessary to do what the seasoned reduced carbohydrate dieters suggest. And remember, this list is not inclusive. These factors are just the ones most commonly cited by reduced carbohydrate dieters. The process of ruling out all the factors that may be slowing your weight loss can take several weeks; it cannot be done in a day or two. This period is usually marked by a great deal of experimentation that will give you a lot of information about your body's response to reduced carbohydrate dieting. Taking the time to walk through all of these possible causes will dramatically increase your chances for success.

4

Take Action

Now that you have learned about the common stumbling blocks that can stall even the dedicated low carbohydrate dieters, it is time to talk about some actions that you can take to make the most of your new eating lifestyle. Experienced low carbohydrate dieters know that it is important not only to overcome obstacles, but also to take proactive steps to maximize success. The focus of this chapter is to provide you with information about the steps you can take to speed your weight loss and overcome stalls and plateaus.

Go Back to the Basics

If you started a reduced carbohydrate diet after hearing about it from a friend or picking up some basic information from a magazine article or web site, do yourself a favor and thoroughly read one of the books on the subject. These books, written by experts with years of experience, fully explain how reduced carbohydrate dieting works. People experienced with the diets know that those who try to "wing it" struggle with truly understanding the diets. This lack of understanding shows in their degree of success; they make some basic mistakes that often have tremendous impact on their rate of weight loss.

If you have already read one of the books, go back and read it again. These books are full of detail, and you may have missed some important points the first time around. Even if you understood everything clearly the first time, you may have forgotten some of the nuances as you settled into your routine. Rereading the book after you have become experienced with the diet can bring a whole new dimension of understanding. It can also help you recapture the spirit that may have helped motivate you in the beginning.

If you have already reread your book, consider reading one of the other titles. Many dieters create their own successful approach by adapting concepts from several of the bestsellers. Although most of the authors are physicians who use reduced carbohydrate dieting to treat their patients, each of them has his or her own distinctive approach. Therefore, you can learn something of value from every book you read. All of the books are available in bookstores, as well as public libraries.

A New Beginning

After refreshing your memory about the basic principles of your diet plan by rereading your book, go back to the fundamentals and begin the program again. For example, if your chosen plan recommends an introduction stage, repeat it. A couple of weeks of practicing the basics can give you some great insights about yourself fairly quickly. For example, if you find that returning to the lowest carbohydrate intake recommended by your plan speeds your weight loss, you probably have been a victim of "carbo creep." Carbo creep occurs when you gradually add "just a little" more carbohydrate until eventually your weight loss slows.

Another great reason to return to the fundamentals of your diet is to find the new level of carbohydrate intake that is low enough to allow you to continue losing weight now that you are smaller and lighter. For example, it takes more energy and more calories to power a 200-pound body than it does a body that weighs 150 pounds. So, as your weight falls, your energy needs also fall, and you may need to reevaluate how much carbohydrate you need to power your body and still lose weight.

Going back to the essentials also allows you to eliminate, all at once, the stumbling blocks discussed in Chapter 3. After spending a couple of weeks eating only the essential foods your plan allows, you can reinstate them one at a time. By adding each item back individually, you can isolate those that are a problem for you. Stagger them by adding just one every two or more weeks, so you can more accurately isolate their effects. For example, if you reintroduce aspartame to your diet and your weight loss once again slows, it is likely that artificial sweeteners are a problem for you.

A word of caution: Resist the temptation to eat "the Last Supper of Carbohydrate" the day before you start over. This will only make it harder for you to get started again, especially if your carbohydrate addiction is haunting you. If breaking your carbohydrate addiction was a significant problem for you at the start of your diet, going back to the fundamentals may be the only way for you to once again gain control over it. Gorging on carbohydrate just before restarting your diet will only serve to strengthen your carbohydrate cravings at a time when you need increased control. And it generates more work for you, as the extra carbohydrate will only serve to build up your glycogen and body fat stores.

Keep a Food Journal

I know there are several of you who groaned inwardly (or perhaps even outwardly) when you read the above heading. Writing down everything you eat seems cumbersome and time-consuming, and wasn't the promise of reduced carbohydrate dieting that we need never obsess about every detail of our diet again? For those who are losing weight slowly or are stuck in a plateau, food diaries are recommended over and over again by seasoned dieters. Many dieters have found keeping a journal to be an eye-opening experience, even if they do it for only a few days. The recipients of this excellent advice who choose to follow it are often shocked by the outcome. They often report that they discovered they were actually taking in many more (or fewer) grams of carbohydrate or calories than they had been estimating—sometimes twice as much or even more. Since the most common causes of slow weight loss are widely believed to be excessive carbohydrate intake or inappropriate calorie or protein intake, the only sure method for determining if this is the case for you is to accurately calculate your daily intake of carbohydrate, calories, and protein.

To begin your journal, for a couple of days (at least), write down everything you eat without making any changes to your usual eating pattern. When I say write down everything, I mean write down *everything*—even that single stray M&M you found in the couch cushions (admit it— we all do it!). Every morsel, including the little bits you taste test while preparing meals, should be included. In the beginning, this may involve measuring and weighing your food to be accurate. Counting everything accurately is important because when a carbohydrate molecule enters your blood, it does not matter if it was part of a nibble or a feast; your body uses it as fuel rather than breaking down your fat stores. We can fool our minds, but we cannot fool our bodies.

Using a good nutrition resource, calculate the calories and grams of carbohydrate and protein for each of the foods you ate and total them for the day. For many people, the reason their weight loss is slow is obvious immediately. Comparing the results to the recommended ranges presented in Chapter 3 can produce quite a shock for some people. For example, one low carbohydrate dieter said, "Holy cow! I ate 3,000 calories and 100 grams of carbohydrate yesterday! No wonder my scale is not moving!" Other people may realize they are eating way below the recommended intake level.

Wendi found that keeping a food journal was well worth her time. On her first day, she was very surprised to realize she took in 54 grams of carbohydrate when she had mentally estimated her intake at less than 30 grams. During her second day, she thought she was doing very well until she discovered her steamed artichoke had 11.9 grams of carbohydrate and the five sticks of gum she chewed had 2 grams each. When she added the carbohydrate from the artificial sweetener, cheese, and eggs she ate, she surprisingly found herself at her maximum daily allotment of carbohydrate by 2:30 in the afternoon.

Food journals can serve other purposes, too. Rather than using it to identify the cause of a slowed loss, you can use it to learn how to make food choices that will allow you to keep your intake within the recommended ranges. For example, Teresa once thought that she could not live without her huge mug (40 ounces) of decaffeinated coffee every morning. But after keeping a food journal for one day, she realized that with the cream and sweetener she was adding to it, she was consuming nearly a third of her daily allotment before 7 A.M. She had to decide whether her beloved coffee was more important to her than the weight loss she was forgoing by drinking it. After evaluating it in this light, she came to realize it simply was not worth it to her and she eliminated it. Most people find that once they bring their carbohydrate, calorie, and protein intake in line with the recommended ranges, their rate of weight loss increases.

For others, the answer may not be so easy or obvious. If your carbohydrate, calorie, and protein counts are within the recommended ranges, you will need to do more work. The source of the problem may be one of the stumbling blocks listed in Chapter 3 rather than your overall intake. If you have friends experienced with the reduced carbohydrate lifestyle, you might find it helpful to get their opinion on the matter. Even better, if you have access to the web, consider posting a day or two of your diary to a reduced carbohydrate support group under their preferred heading. It is common for groups to use a heading such as "Attention: Carb Detectives" (or something similar) to alert the participants that a dieter needs help. The group participants will review the content of the food diary and offer advice to help ferret out the possible stumbling blocks. By viewing your actual intake, they are in a much better position to offer suggestions that may help speed your weight loss.

Be a Detective

For a food journal to be a truly effective tool, it must be accurate. Therefore, you must know the nutritional values of all the foods you are eating. At a minimum, you should invest in a good nutritional reference. Many are available in book form, while others are available in computer software. Whichever format you choose, be sure to get one that contains more than just the carbohydrate count. It should also list the calorie and protein counts of common foods. If you are following a plan that allows subtracting the fiber count from the total carbohydrate count, you will need a resource that also lists the fiber counts.

The advantage of books is that they are usually cheaper and more portable. The advantage of computer software is that most programs also perform a variety of nutritional analyses and generate graphs and pie charts. They also require very little math skill on the user's part. Not all of them are expensive. One package that can be found at office supply stores sells for approximately $10. If you cook a lot, it might also be worth investing in cookbook software that will calculate the nutritional values of your favorite recipes.

For information on foods not listed in these commonly available resources, the USDA has an excellent free database at its official web site. The address is http://www.nal.usda.gov/fnic/cgi-bin/nut_search.pl. This site is particularly helpful in finding nutritional values for unusual foods such as spices and wild game. For example, one dieter who lives in Alaska was able to find the nutritional values for caribou—raw, cooked, and roasted—at this site!

And don't forget to be vigilant about uncovering hidden carbohydrate in your food. As discussed in Chapter 3, you should not simply accept a nutritional value of 0 grams for the carbohydrate in prepared foods. Be sure to follow the techniques given to determine if a food contains hidden carbohydrate, and if it does, attribute it with at least 0.5

gram of carbohydrate per serving in your daily totals. In addition, be sure to look up all the foods you eat to minimize your chance of overlooking sources of carbohydrate. Overlooked carbohydrate includes bread fillers and other recipe ingredients (especially in restaurant food). Also check the carbohydrate in the medications and supplements you are taking, and count them in the total, too.

Some people find a food journal to be so valuable that they continue to keep it for a long time. Other people find it useful only until they develop a new routine that speeds their weight loss. They resume keeping a journal only when their weight loss slows or they once again reach a plateau.

Adjust Your Intake as Your Weight Falls

It is a common perception among seasoned reduced carbohydrate dieters that weight loss appears to slow as you approach your goal weight. As discussed in Chapter 2, this may be only a problem of perception, and weight loss may not have slowed at all. For example, if a woman weighed 200 pounds and lost 1 percent of her body weight per week, she would be losing 2 pounds per week. When her weight fell to 150 pounds, she might still be losing 1 percent of her body weight per week, but this would equate to only 1.5 pounds per week. If this woman looked only at the number of pounds she lost, she would mistakenly conclude that her weight loss had slowed down.

If you are losing the same percentage of your body weight each week, or if your loss is varying only slightly, you probably do not need to adjust your food intake. On the other hand, if your weight loss is truly slowing, as evidenced by a drop in the percentage of body weight you are losing per week, you will need to do some work. Take a fresh look at the number of grams of carbohydrate you can eat and still lose weight. You may have to lower your carbohydrate intake to continue losing weight now that you are smaller and lighter. For example, a woman who weighs 200 pounds at the start of her diet may be able to consume 60 grams of carbohydrate per day and lose weight at a satisfactory rate. But, as her weight drops, her weight loss may slow considerably and eventually even reach a plateau. The woman should go back to her plan's lowest recommended carbohydrate intake for a couple of weeks, then gradually reintroduce more carbohydrate into her diet to learn her new acceptable level of carbohydrate intake. (The common recommendation is to add no more than 5 grams of carbohydrate per day until weight loss stops and then retreat slightly to a lower level.) By going through this process again, the woman may find that since she now weighs 50 pounds less, she can take in only 50 grams of carbohydrate per day and continue to lose weight.

You may also have to readjust your calorie intake as your weight falls. As discussed in Chapter 3, the recommended intake is 10 to 12 calories per pound of body weight per day. When the woman in the example above weighed 200 pounds, she might have been able to consume 2,000 to 2,400 calories per day and lose weight. However, once she weighs only 150 pounds, her range shifts downward. She may find that she is now able to take in only 1,500 to 1,800 calories per day and still lose weight.

Plan Ahead

If your food journal reveals that the most likely cause of your slow weight loss is too much carbohydrate, you must develop strategies to reduce your carbohydrate intake to a level that will allow you to lose weight more quickly. For many people, especially those who work outside the home, that can take quite a bit of planning. Our world is abundant with foods that are low in fat and high in carbohydrate, and we must learn how to live comfortably in it. Unfortunately, reduced carbohydrate dieters learn very quickly that this is not an easy task, as there are very few commercial, convenient foods that are low in carbohydrate. Vending machines and convenience stores overflow with high carbohydrate treats. Nuts and pork rinds are about the only low carbohydrate options, and nuts must be limited due to their calorie counts. Fast-food restaurants present the same dilemma. You can eat a cheeseburger without the bun for only so long! Even worse, restaurants have adopted the irritating practice of adding sugar to recipes and foods that would otherwise be suitable, such as creamy salad dressings.

Most of us find that we must be creative and plan ahead to resist the temptation of easy high carbohydrate foods. Charlene is a good example of how advance preparation can carry you safely through a strong temptation. Charlene was scheduled to go out to dinner with her friends to celebrate a job promotion for one of them. As bad luck would have it, the guest of honor had chosen Charlene's favorite Italian restaurant for the celebration. Knowing that this group of friends was very likely to indulge in desserts, Charlene made a low carbohydrate chocolate cheesecake before leaving her home.

Charlene was quite relieved to find that one of the specials for the evening was grilled swordfish, and with a quick substitution of steamed broccoli for the pasta that usually accompanied the fish, she kept well within her limits and had a great low carbohydrate meal. Feeling as though she had dodged a bullet, she relaxed. But, as she had expected, the worst was yet to come. True to form, every one of her comrades chose to order a decadent chocolate dessert. Charlene recalls that it took every ounce of strength she had not to order the dessert, too. She says the only way she got through it was by reminding herself of the cheesecake that was waiting for her at home in her refrigerator. She said she was so consumed with the thought of the cheesecake that when she got home, she headed straight for the kitchen. Although she ate much more of it than she would have otherwise, planning ahead certainly saved her from the restaurant dessert that would have spelled disaster.

The following ideas from seasoned reduced carbohydrate dieters should help you control your carbohydrate intake in a world of easily available high carbohydrate foods.

- For many of us, reduced carbohydrate dieting means that we must learn how to cook. Simply living off convenience foods and restaurant meals does not work. Until the world is more hospitable to reduced carbohydrate dieting, we are obliged to create our own menus in our own homes. (By the way, restaurants specializing in reduced carbohydrate meals are opening in some cities.) Preparing your own food grants you more control and allows you to be certain of the ingredients in the dish. By doing your own cooking, you are much less likely to eat hidden or overlooked carbohydrate.
- Use your new cooking skills to prepare meals in advance as much as possible. By preparing meals ahead of time and freezing them, you can make your own convenience foods. The only difference is that your meals are your own creations rather than the creations of the food industry.

- Keep acceptable foods on hand for those times you need to eat something quickly. For example, stash away a few low carbohydrate protein bars (if glycerine does not stall your weight loss). Other good foods are hard-boiled or deviled eggs, string cheese, celery with cream cheese, meat and cheese roll-ups, nuts, crispy bacon strips, pepperoni slices, and high fiber, low carbohydrate crackers.

- If you work outside your home, take your lunch to work with you and keep a supply of homemade snacks and other low carbohydrate foods on hand. There is nothing worse than the siren song of the vending machine during that mid-afternoon slump that many of us get at work.

- Empty your cupboards as much as possible of foods that do not fit your reduced carbohydrate lifestyle. If you live alone or with another reduced carbohydrate dieter, this means that *all* carbohydrate-laden foods must go. If you live with people who are normal weighted and protest the idea of giving up their favorite foods for *your* diet, at least separate them from your stock of low carbohydrate foods. One mother said that she took all of her children's treats and placed them in a separate cupboard. She avoids that cupboard so she does not have to see them every time she goes to her pantry. She also purchased a lockbox for her family's chocolate candy (her greatest weakness). By giving the only keys to her husband, she was able to dramatically lower the number of times she took "just a bite."

- When you go to a party, take your favorite low carbohydrate treat with you. Knowing that you have a scrumptious alternative can be just the thing you need to get you safely through the maze of high carbohydrate foods that are bound to be there.

- When eating out, request that your meal be modified to fit your new lifestyle. For example, a popular reduced carbohydrate request is for the inside of a bagel to be scooped out (forming a little round moat of sorts) and filled with cream cheese.

With a little bit of planning, some foresight, and a lot of experience, you can lower your total carbohydrate count despite the overwhelming presence of carbohydrate-rich foods.

Use the Glycemic Index

As discussed in Chapter 3, many reduced carbohydrate dieters have learned that simple, refined sources of carbohydrate have much more "fattening power" than do unrefined, complex sources of carbohydrate. Simple, refined carbohydrate enters the blood more quickly, raises the blood glucose levels higher, triggers larger insulin releases, and, slows weight loss.

Many experienced dieters use a popular system for choosing complex, unrefined sources of carbohydrate and avoiding simple, refined sources of carbohydrate. This system is known as the glycemic index, and its use is advocated by several of the reduced carbohydrate diet experts. (Note that the authors of *Protein Power* do not support its use.) The glycemic index is a rating system that ranks foods according to their effect on the level of glucose in the blood. Originally developed to guide diabetics in their food choices, the glycemic index is also helpful for reduced carbohydrate dieters.

The foods included in the glycemic index were tested and ranked according to their effect on the blood glucose levels two to three hours after being eaten. The ones that cause a rapid and marked rise in the blood sugar levels have high glycemic index value. These foods are generally considered to be undesirable sources of carbohydrate. Examples are foods that contain simple, refined carbohydrate such as white bread, table sugar, pasta, and potatoes.

On the other hand, foods that have slower and less dramatic effects on the blood glucose levels have low glycemic index values. These foods are generally considered to be more desirable. They include high fiber, unprocessed, natural foods such as whole, fresh vegetables.

If you are interested in learning more about the glycemic index, see Chapter 6 for a list of resources.

Eat More Fiber

Given the undeserved reputation of the reduced carbohydrate diet as being a meat-and-cheese-only diet, many people are surprised to learn that the consumption of high fiber foods such as vegetables is not only acceptable, but actively encouraged. Low carbohydrate, high fiber foods are helpful in speeding weight loss in a couple of ways. First, the fiber in the foods cannot be broken down by our digestive system. Therefore, it passes through largely undigested. Because the fiber cannot be digested, the other components of the food, including the carbohydrate, are digested more slowly. This causes the level of glucose in our blood to rise more slowly, which, in turn, causes less insulin to be produced in response. Because less insulin is released, the blood glucose levels remain even, and hypoglycemia (low blood glucose) does not develop. So, the first reason eating foods with fiber leads us to eat less food overall is that the carbohydrate in the food is released into the bloodstream slowly and evenly. You reap the benefits of stabilized blood glucose levels by being less hungry and having fewer and less intense carbohydrate cravings. Therefore, you eat less.

The second reason eating high fiber foods leads us to eat less food is that since it takes longer for our digestive systems to break down fiber, it allows us to feel fuller longer. Thus, we eat less, and our total calorie and carbohydrate intake falls. If you reviewed your food journal and learned that the most likely cause of your slow weight loss is either too many calories or too much carbohydrate, increasing your fiber intake can be an effective strategy for lowering both.

Because the fiber in food cannot be digested and it also slows the digestion of other food components, reduced carbohydrate dieters often use the easy technique of subtracting a food's fiber count from its carbohydrate count to estimate its power to raise the blood glucose levels. This technique is taken from *Protein Power*, although other reduced carbohydrate diet book authors support it. The principle is simple: The higher the fiber count in a food, the slower the food will be digested. Since the fiber in foods cannot be digested, it need not be counted in our total carbohydrate counts (this is the great part). Therefore, we can subtract the fiber count from the total carbohydrate count and include only the difference—the carbohydrate that can be digested—in our daily carbohydrate counts. This method allows us to quickly estimate the power of a food to raise our blood sugar levels, by simply looking at its Nutrition Facts label, and prevents us from overstating our total carbohydrate count.

Eat More Vegetables

When it comes to foods that are naturally low in carbohydrate and high in fiber, vegetables are king. For example, Figure 4.1 shows a label from a can of French-cut green beans.

By reading the label, we learn that the green beans have a total carbohydrate count of 4 grams per half-cup serving, which lets us know right away that this is a low carbohydrate food. By looking further, we see that the carbohydrate total is made up of 2 grams of fiber and 2 grams of sugar, letting us know that this is a relatively high fiber food. Using the recommended technique, we subtract the 2 grams of fiber from the 4 grams of total carbohydrate, leaving only 2 grams of digestible carbohydrate. Therefore, we can quickly estimate that this food is unlikely to cause a surge in our blood sugar levels or in our insulin re-

Nutrition Facts

Serving Size ½ cup (120g)
Servings Per Container About 3

Amount Per Serving	
Calories 20	**Calories from Fat** 0
	% Daily Value*
Total Fat <1g	0%
Saturated Fat 0g	0%
Cholesterol 0mg	0%
Sodium 400mg	17%
Total Carbohydrate 4g	1%
Dietary Fiber 2g	8%
Sugars 2g	
Protein <1g	Not a significant source of protein

Vitamin A	4%	Vitamin C	4%
Calcium	2%	Iron	0%

*Percent Daily Values are based on a 2,000 calorie diet.

INGREDIENTS: Green Beans, Water, and Salt.

Figure 4.1. This label off a can of green beans shows the vegetable is a good high-fiber choice.

leases. Therefore, we count only 2 grams of carbohydrate in our food journal.

To verify that this Nutrition Facts label checks out, we should quickly analyze its contents. The product has 4 grams of carbohydrate per serving, accounting for 16 of the 20 calories. The protein count is listed as less than 1 gram per serving, so if we estimate each serving has 0.5 gram of protein, we would have 2 more calories. The fat content is also listed as less than 1 gram per serving, so if we estimate each serving has 0.5 gram of fat, we would have another 4 calories bringing our total to 22 calories per serving, which is very close to the rounded count of 20 on the label. This analysis verifies the relative accuracy of the label and explains why green beans are one of the favorite vegetables of reduced carbohydrate dieters: They are low in carbohydrate, are high in fiber, and taste great with butter.

A word of caution: Some manufacturers beat us to the punch and do not include the fiber count in the total carbohydrate count on the Nutrition Facts label. Be suspicious of any label on which the total carbohydrate count minus the fiber count results in a digestible carbohydrate count of 0 (or close to it). If you are suspicious, perform a label analysis to see if the calories add up. For example, Celia purchased a brand of crispbread that had a very confusing label. The label said the crispbread had 2.4 grams of total carbohydrate and 3.5 grams of fiber. This results in a negative digestive carbohydrate count. Obviously, this manufacturer had already subtracted the fiber count from the total carbohydrate count. To estimate this product's true nutritional content, Celia had to consult an independent nutritional reference source.

Other great low carbohydrate foods frequently enjoyed by reduced carbohydrate dieters are listed in Table 4.1.

Table 4.1. Good low carbohydrate foods for reduced carbohydrate dieters.

Food (1/2 cup unless otherwise stated)	Total Carbohydrate (in grams)	Fiber (in grams)	Digestible Carbohydrate (in grams)
Mustard greens, boiled, drained	1.5	1.4	0.1
Alfalfa seed sprouts, raw	0.6	0.4	0.2
Lettuce, looseleaf, shredded	1.0	0.5	0.5
Bamboo shoots, boiled, drained	1.2	0.6	0.6
Turnip greens, boiled, drained	3.1	2.5	0.6
Turnip, boiled, drained, mashed	5.6	2.3	0.9
Broccoli*, raw, chopped	2.3	1.3	1.0
Cucumber, raw, sliced, with peel	1.4	0.4	1.0
Zucchini, raw, sliced	1.7	0.7	1.0
Mushrooms, raw, pieces	1.4	0.4	1.0
Olives, ripe, 1 oz.	2.0	1.0	1.0
Spinach, boiled, drained	3.4	2.2	1.2
Celery, raw, diced	2.2	1.0	1.2
Radish, raw, sliced	2.1	0.9	1.2
Cauliflower, raw, 1" pieces	2.6	1.3	1.3
Avocado*, raw, trimmed	5.5	3.8	1.5
Cabbage, shredded, boiled, drained	3.3	1.7	1.6
Eggplant, 1" cubes, boiled, drained	3.2	1.2	2.0
Collard greens, boiled, drained	4.7	2.7	2.0
Asparagus, cut, boiled, drained	3.8	1.4	2.4
Squash, summer, boiled, drained	3.9	1.3	2.6
Green beans, boiled, drained	4.9	2.0	2.9
Tomato*, chopped	4.2	1.0	3.2
Sweet red pepper, raw, chopped	4.8	1.5	3.3
Snow pea pods*, boiled, drained	5.7	2.2	3.5
Pumpkin, boiled, drained, mashed	6.0	1.4	4.6
Brussels sprouts*, boiled, drained	6.8	2.0	4.8
Artichoke heart*, boiled	9.4	4.5	4.9

* These vegetables are limited in *The Carbohydrate Addict's Diet* to Reward Meals only.

Source: USDA Nutrient Database for Standard Reference.

The foods in the table are fresh (not canned) and ranked according to their digestible carbohydrate count.

Another reason to include more vegetables in your diet is that they provide variety. Food boredom is often cited as a reason dieters resort to eating "off-plan" foods. If you do not like the low carbohydrate vegetables, you should invest in one of the many popular low carbohydrate cookbooks or visit the low carbohydrate web sites to get tasty recipes. Many dieters report that once they became aware of the creative ways to cook low carbohydrate vegetables, they began to eat more of them.

For example, Maria rediscovered pesto sauce. For years, she ignored pesto and similar sauces because they did not fit into her low fat diet. For the first few months of low carbohydrate dieting, she did not consider them simply because she had become so accustomed to ignoring them at the grocery store. By luck, she found a brand that had only 2 grams of carbohydrate per 0.25-cup serving and, suddenly, she found she had new options for cooking vegetables. She discovered she could increase her vegetable intake much more easily when they were accented with pesto or other enjoyable low carbohydrate sauces.

Eat Other Sources of Fiber

In addition to vegetables, nuts are a favorite food among reduced carbohydrate dieters. They are low in carbohydrate and high in fiber, making them a great snack food. Macadamias are king, with the lowest digestible carbohydrate count of all the popular varieties. Other good selections are brazil nuts and almonds. On the other hand, some varieties, such as cashews, are denser in carbohydrate and should be eaten sparingly. Also, while many nuts are low in digestible carbohydrate, they are calorie-dense, and the calories can add up quickly. If you find that your slow weight loss is most likely caused by an overabundance of calories, you should limit your intake of nuts. Table 4.2 lists common varieties of nuts and gives their digestible carbohydrate count.

There are also a few fruits that can fit into your reduced carbohydrate diet, presented in Table 4.3. While some of these foods are higher in digestible carbohydrate than most vegetables and should be eaten in moderation, they can help squelch carbohydrate cravings. A serving of artificially sweetened raspberries is a much better snack than a bag of cookies when strong carbohydrate cravings strike.

Table 4.2. Nuts and their digestible carbohydrate counts.

Nuts and Seeds (1 oz. shelled unless otherwise stated)	Total Carbohydrate (in grams)	Fiber (in grams)	Digestible Carbohydrate (in grams)
Pecans, dry roasted	3.8	2.7	1.1
Macadamias, dry roasted	3.8	2.3	1.5
Brazil nuts, dried, unbalanced	3.6	1.5	1.9
Black walnuts, dried	3.4	1.4	2.0
Almonds, dry roasted	5.5	3.3	2.2
Hazelnuts (filberts), dry roasted	5.0	2.7	2.3
Sesame seeds, shelled, roasted	7.3	4.0	3.3
Peanuts, dry roasted	6.0	2.3	3.7
Sunflower seeds, kernels, dry roasted	6.8	3.1	3.7
Mixed nuts with peanuts, dry roasted	7.2	2.6	4.6
Pistachios, dry roasted	7.9	2.9	5.0
Pumpkin seeds, including the shell, raw	15.3	10.2	5.1
Cashews, dry roasted	9.3	0.9	8.4

Source: USDA Nutrient Database for Standard Reference.

Table 4.3. Fruits and their digestible carbohydrate counts.

Fresh Fruit (1/2 cup unless otherwise noted)	Total Carbohydrate (in grams)	Fiber (in grams)	Digestible Carbohydrate (in grams)
Raspberries	7.1	4.2	2.9
Strawberries	5.2	1.7	3.5
Cranberries, whole	6.0	2.0	4.0
Blackberries	9.2	3.6	5.6
Cantaloupe	6.7	0.6	6.1

Source: USDA Nutrient Database for Standard Reference.

Surprisingly, there are some high fiber, reduced calorie breads that can be incorporated into most reduced carbohydrate diet plans, as shown in Table 4.4. As the reduced carbohydrate lifestyle gains momentum, mainstream bakeries are beginning to respond by producing reduced carbohydrate breads. I found four at my local grocery store that have digestible carbohydrate counts under 8 grams per slice. One of them has only 5 grams per slice. Each of these breads is a full slice of bread, not the thin sliced version that is common among reduced calorie breads. In addition to reduced carbohydrate breads, whole-grain crispbreads (thin, crisp, crackerlike breads) are very popular among reduced carbohydrate dieters because they contain only 5 to 6 grams of digestible carbohydrate per 2.5-inch by 5.5-inch slice.

Consider Fiber Supplements

Many reduced carbohydrate dieters who find they have difficulty incorporating significant amounts of fiber into their diets by eating whole, natural foods turn to fiber supplements to do the job. They claim that when they take fiber supplements immediately prior to meals, along with

Table 4.4. Reduced carbohydrate breads and their digestible carbohydrate counts.

Bread (1 slice unless otherwise noted)	Total Carbohydrate (in grams)	Fiber (in grams)	Digestible Carbohydrate (in grams)
Healthy Life, 100% Whole Wheat Bread	8.0	3.0	5.0
Wonder Light, Reduced Calorie Wheat	9.0	2.5	6.5
Roman Meal Light, Wheat	10.0	3.0	7.0
Pepperidge Farm, Light Style, Wheat	9.0	1.0	8.0
WASA Light Rye Crispbread	6.0	1.0	5.0
WASA Sourdough Rye Crispbread	7.0	1.0	6.0

Source: Manufacturer Nutrition Facts labels.

meals, or between meals, they not only eat less, but are much less hungry overall.

Fortunately, there has been a proliferation of fiber products available at pharmacies and supermarkets in the past several years. While nearly all of them are derived from psyllium husks (the husks of a natural grain), some come from other sources. They also come in several forms, including powders to be mixed with water, gelatins that can be diluted with water or eaten directly, granules and tablets that can simply be swallowed, tablets that can be chewed, snack bars that can be eaten on the go, and crackers.

Words of caution: First, several fiber preparations include significant amounts of sugar and other sources of hidden carbohydrate. Some of them have Nutrition Facts labels that clearly provide the carbohydrate and fiber counts, but not all do, since they are not required to. If the product does not have a Nutrition Facts label, you must estimate the carbohydrate content based on the active and inactive ingredients lists. Look for varieties that are either unsweetened or artificially sweetened, which usually have Nutrition Facts labels because they are often marketed to diabetics. Second, watch out for fiber preparations that have laxatives added to them. Laxatives are habit forming, sometimes in as little as a few days. Therefore, fiber products that have added laxatives should be avoided. Third, if you are not accustomed to eating significant amounts of fiber, increase your fiber intake slowly. Our bowels have "stretch receptors" that cause pain when the bowel is suddenly stretched beyond its usual capacity. Therefore, suddenly increasing the amount of fiber bulk you eat could be quite uncomfortable. Fourth, fiber supplements should not be routinely used as a substitute for high fiber vegetables. While they provide important fiber, they do not provide the vitamins and other nutrients that vegetables do.

Get to Know Your Natural Grocer

Natural food grocery stores carry several foods that are low in carbohydrate and high in fiber that are not readily available in conventional grocery stores. These "natural foods" are often organic, low in sugar, made from whole grain, high in fiber, and minimally refined. For example, I visited my favorite natural food grocer and found the foods listed in Table 4.5. While some of these products may be an acquired taste, some are little jewels. (I especially love soy nuts.)

Table 4.5. "Natural foods" and their digestible carbohydrate counts.

Food	Total Carbohydrate (in grams)	Fiber (in grams)	Digestible Carbohydrate (in grams)
Flaxseed meal (flour substitute)*, 1/4 cup	8.0	8.0	0
Cream-cheese-style soy, 1/4 cup	0	0	0
Baba ganoush (eggplant and tahini spread), 2 tbs.	2.0	1.0	1.0
Garlic and peppercorn salad dressing, 2 tbs.	1.6	0.2	1.4
Soy nuts (roasted soybeans), 1/4 cup	8.0	6.0	2.0
Pumpkorn (seasoned pumpkin seeds), 1/3 cup	4.0	2.0	2.0
Miso-Cup (vegetable soup broth), 1 cup	3.0	<1	2.0
Macadamia butter (nut butter), 2 tbs.	5.0	3.0	2.0
Eggplant meze (spicy spreadable eggplant), 2 tbs.	2.0	0	2.0
Almond butter, 2 tbs.	6.0	3.0	3.0
Smoked pasilla (spicy salsa), 2 tbs.	3.0	0	3.0
Bran-a-Crisp Fiber Crackers, 1 cracker	6.0	2.0	4.0
Pistachio butter, 2 tbs.	9.0	4.0	5.0

*This product claims to be made from 100% whole grain fiber.

Source: Manufacturer Nutrition Facts labels.

Drink Plenty of Water

Drinking plenty of water has long been recommended by diet experts for people on any kind of diet. Reduced carbohydrate dieters agree that it works and works well. If you have not done so already, you should become a member of the "glub club." When it comes to increasing weight loss and breaking stalls and plateaus, the importance of adequate water intake cannot be overstated. Many reduced carbohydrate dieters say that the amount of weight they lose is directly proportional to the amount of water they drink: The more they drink, the more they lose. In fact, many people report their weight loss stalled for no other reason than not drinking enough water.

The most frequently cited reason adequate water intake is beneficial is that it keeps you well hydrated. Hydration is important for all dieters, but it is of extra benefit to reduced carbohydrate dieters. One of the effects of reduced carbohydrate dieting is that it has a natural diuretic effect; our bodies do not hold water as readily. As a result, we risk dehydration if we do not take in enough water to replace the water that we lose. Dehydration can lead to overeating for some dieters because they may misinterpret thirst as hunger and react by eating rather than drinking. Drinking enough water prevents this misunderstanding and, therefore, can decrease overall food intake.

If you are on a ketogenic diet, water is important for flushing ketones from your body. The authors of *Protein Power* state that water actually promotes weight loss on ketogenic diets by flushing ketone bodies from the bloodstream. They theorize that drinking a lot of water reduces the number of ketone bodies available for the body to use as fuel. Therefore, the body must break down more fat to produce more ketone bodies for fuel and more fat loss occurs. In other words, if there is a high level of ketones in the blood, the body will not break down fat stores to produce more ketone bodies. Drinking a lot of water will keep the level of ketone bodies lower and, therefore, will increase and speed up weight loss.

Effects on Ketostix Reactions

People who are on ketogenic diets find that as their water intake increases, the degree of their Ketostix urine testing strip reaction decreases. In other words, the Ketostix test strip becomes a lighter color of pink. Unfortunately, these folks often misinterpret the lighter readings to mean that they are losing weight more slowly when, in fact, this may not be true. Seasoned low carbohydrate dieters know there is a weak correlation between the degree of darkness of the Ketostix and the rate of fat loss. The degree of darkness tells you only two things: whether or not you are in ketosis, and the degree of concentration of ketone bodies in your urine, not in your blood. Therefore, it is important to clearly understand that the concentration of the ketone bodies in your urine is directly affected by the amount of water you drink.

An easy way to think of this dynamic is to substitute salt-water. If you were to dissolve a tablespoon of salt in a cup of water and taste it, your taste buds would react strongly because many salt molecules would fall on your tongue with each sip. In contrast, if you were to add a tablespoon of salt to a larger amount of water—let's say a gallon—your taste buds would react less strongly because fewer salt molecules would hit your tongue. While the total amount of salt added to the water is the same in both examples, how your tongue reacts to it is different because one solution is concentrated while the other is diluted.

The same is true of ketone bodies. When we drink a small amount of water, the number of ketone bodies that fall on the Ketostix pad is greater because the urine is concentrated. Therefore, the reaction is a deep purple. After drinking more water, the same number of ketone bodies is spread out in more urine. Therefore, fewer of them will strike the Ketostix pad and a lighter reaction will occur (usually pink). In both examples, the number of ketone bodies the body is producing remains the same. Therefore, the rate of fat loss is the same—only the reaction of the Ketostix changes.

It is common for new low carbohydrate dieters who are inexperienced at using Ketostix to become unduly concerned with the lighter reaction. Sharon sought help from her fellow low carbohydrate dieters because she believed the diet was not working for her. She was not gauging her success by how much weight she was losing or how much better her clothes were fitting. Rather, she was concerned because she was not able to achieve a deep purple reaction on her Ketostix. She was drinking ten glasses of water per day. She learned from her peers that it is normal for Ketostix to be lighter in color when urine is diluted. Her peers also gently reminded her that she was getting her goals a bit confused. The goal of the diet is to lose fat, not to achieve Ketostix glory. She learned she should not be concerned with the degree of the Ketostix reaction; she should be concerned only with losing body fat.

How Much to Drink

The general rule of thumb that many seasoned low carbohydrate dieters follow is to base the amount of water to drink on the amount of weight to be lost. People with normal kidney function should drink at least 64 ounces of water per day, plus an additional 8 ounces for each 25 pounds of weight they need to lose. For example, if a man weighs 220 pounds and has a goal of losing 50 pounds to bring him down to around 170 pounds, he should drink 64 ounces plus 16 ounces for a total of 80 ounces of water per day. A simpler recommendation is to take half your body weight in pounds and drink that amount of water in ounces per day. Using this approach, this same 220-pound man would drink 110 ounces of water each day.

If you are on a ketogenic diet, you should drink enough water to keep the degree of your Ketostix reaction at a light to moderate level. A dark purple reaction is considered a clear indication that you are not drinking enough water to be well hydrated. Another good gauge of whether you are drinking enough water is the degree of comfort of your mouth. You should drink enough water to keep the uncomfortable mouth sensations that commonly accompany ketosis to a minimum.

New dieters often balk at drinking this much water, especially if they are very overweight. They protest that to drink that much water, they must take up residence in the bathroom, and at first they do! But over time, sometimes in as little as a few days, the body adjusts to consuming this much water, and the trips to the bathroom become much less frequent. If you have an outside job or are in an environment in which frequent trips to the bathroom are disruptive, you may wish to increase your water intake by adding just a glass per day until you reach your recommended amount. This allows your body to gradually adjust. However, if you choose to jump right in and increase your water intake all at once, you should probably do so on a day when you can hang around the house. It is not a good idea to suddenly begin drinking a lot more water on a day when you are in very long meetings or on a long hike!

What to Drink

The most passionate water drinkers often insist that when they say "water," they mean water. Others who are less devoted to pure water say anything that is a fluid at room temperature can be counted. Most people are in the middle of the road and say that water-based drinks that do not contain calories or carbohydrate (that leaves out coffee) can be counted as water. They point out that many people cannot stand to drink a great deal of water and, rather than forcing it down or going without it altogether, feel it is better to drink other water-based fluids. There is, however, almost universal agreement that carbonated sodas should not be counted toward the total water count because of all the additives they contain. As discussed in Chapter 3, sodas and many other soft drinks contain ingredients that often contribute to stalls, such as caffeine and artificial sweeteners. Drinking water in their place will avoid these potential problems.

At a minimum, you should increase your fluid intake until your rate of weight loss increases. You should also consider taking the purists' advice and drink as much of your fluids in the form of water as possible. If you cannot stand water, following are some ideas from seasoned reduced carbohydrate dieters that may help you drink more:

- Precede the water with something very spicy, such as barbecue-flavored nuts, peppers, or Tabasco sauce. Norman suggests preceding the water with something salty and crunchy. He recommends salted, roasted almonds.
- Drink water when you are hungry. Some people report that being hungry improves the taste of water and it seems to go down easier. And drinking water before meals has the added benefit of filling your stomach, so you may eat less.
- Dilute tea and other drinks with extra water. For example, if you are eating out and order a glass of iced tea, order a glass of water to go with it. After about a third of your tea is gone, dilute it with water rather than adding more tea to it. This method can easily add 8 ounces or more of water to your daily intake.
- Experiment with bottled water to see if there is a brand you like better. Many people report that they can perceive a taste difference between brands.

- Consider investing in a home water filter or purification system to improve the taste of your tap water. Overall, it can be cheaper than purchasing bottled water.

- Find your preferred water temperature. Many people say they can drink water only if it is at a pleasing temperature. For example, Steve can drink large amounts of water, but it must be cold for him to tolerate it. This is a significant challenge for him because he has an outdoor job in a warm climate. Each night, he fills four large bottles with water and places them in the freezer. Each day, he drinks the water as the ice melts. Others say they can tolerate water much better if it is at room temperature because they dislike the drop in body temperature that cold water causes.

- Drink your total water allotment in several sessions. Linda says she can drink large amounts of water only through a divide-and-conquer approach. She blocks out times when she must drink a certain amount of water. For example, she will drink 12 ounces every even-numbered hour. By the end of the day, she has consumed the 72 ounces she needs. Nancy has a slightly different approach in that she drinks 20 ounces each at breakfast, lunch, and dinner, and 20 ounces more in the evening to get her total 80 ounces.

- Drink your water through a straw. Many people report that this helps a great deal.

- Find a fun, creative way to keep track of how much water you drink. Ed's goal is to drink 80 ounces of water a day. Each morning he places ten pennies in his left pocket, and each time he drinks an 8-ounce glass of water, he moves one penny from his left pocket to his right. He can do a quick check to review his progress toward his goal any time of the day simply by checking his pockets.

- Drink non-flavored carbonated water. Jennie says she does not enjoy drinking water and really misses soda at times. She found a solution by drinking non-flavored carbonated water, such as club soda. For her, club soda is a good substitute when her soda cravings are strong.
- Give it some time. Nearly all reduced carbohydrate dieters who drink the recommended amount of water say they had to overcome an initial resistance. They report that after a few days or weeks, drinking large amounts of water became second nature to them, and they miss it if they are not able to do so.

A word of caution: When you begin to drink more water, you may find that it has a negative impact on your scale weight. If you are dehydrated, either from not taking in enough water or from the diuretic effect of your diet, your scale weight may increase slightly at first. This effect occurs as your body soaks up the water it was missing. As discussed in Chapter 2, water is heavy: it weighs approximately "a pound per pint." This rule of thumb means that if your body absorbs a pint of water, it will add a pound of weight on the scale.

A second word of caution: If you have any medical condition or illness, especially if you have an illness or take medication that impairs your kidney function, you should consult your physician to determine how much water is safe and appropriate for you to drink. Hyponatremia (too little sodium in the blood) is a condition that can occur for some people who drink large amounts of water every day. It is very rare in the United States because we eat much more sodium than is necessary, but it can occur if you are taking certain medications or are on a sodium-restricted diet.

Add Some Exercise

Many people find they are able to successfully lose weight on reduced carbohydrate diets without doing any exercise—a benefit they treasure! However, there is no debate among seasoned reduced carbohydrate dieters that exercise provides an edge in losing fat. We burn energy while doing it, and the "after-burner" effects can last for hours. Exercise adds muscle, which gives our metabolisms a big boost. In fact, estimates are that a pound of muscle burns 35 to 50 calories a day, while a pound of fat burns only about 2 calories per day. Legions of books and magazine articles are devoted to the benefits of exercise, and you should familiarize yourself with them. While most of the exercise advice given in these books and magazines is directly applicable to us, there are some nuances that seasoned reduced carbohydrate dieters have learned over time.

Benefits of Exercise

One of the most helpful benefits of exercise is that it allows us to consume slightly more carbohydrate and still lose weight on the days we exercise. One woman comments that exercise is the price she pays to buy extra diet freedom when she feels an urge to splurge. Rather than denying herself totally, she adds exercise to cover the additional intake. This technique is a godsend on the days we experience increased hunger and carbohydrate cravings. As already discussed, increased hunger is common for women at certain points in their menstrual cycles and for anyone immediately before a whoosh. Rather than battling the hunger, performing mild to moderate exercise is a very healthy way to compensate for the increased intake.

People on ketogenic diets find they get immediate visual feedback that exercise really does work. These people report that almost immediately after mild to moderate exercise, their ketosis deepens for several hours. This visual verification alone is enough to motivate many people to exercise regularly. An added benefit is that as their level of ketosis deepens, their appetite decreases. They use exercise as a tool to curb their appetite on days that hunger is a greater challenge.

Whether or not you are on a ketogenic diet, using exercise to manage your hunger is a very healthy technique, if you do not carry it to an extreme. A word of caution: Never use strenuous exercise as a justification for gorging on carbohydrate. This practice is strongly discouraged because it can be harmful. In addition, do not use strenuous exercise as a method to depress your appetite to the point where you are severely restricting your intake. As discussed in Chapter 3, this is counterproductive.

Further, the authors of *Sugar Busters!* caution that too much exercise can rapidly deplete available energy stores and force the body to convert protein to glucose for fuel. In other words, if you exercise too much too soon and you restrict your intake too much at the same time, your body will use glucogenesis to provide fuel to your body rather than using your fat stores to do it. Proponents of this theory point out that it is supported by reports from people who noticed that their ketosis disappeared rather than increased after strenuous exercise.

While there are many good reasons to add exercise to your life, the really great thing is that it is a wonderful way to break through a plateau. Revving up your metabolism is an excellent way to increase the rate at which your body breaks down fat. Remember Mara, the woman in Chapter

2 who was inspired after graphing her weight loss results over a 23-month period? She also noticed the impact that exercise had on her weight loss. During a three-month period, she frequented her gym consistently five days per week. During those three months, her weight loss averaged nearly 3.75 pounds per week. During the other 20 months, she visited the gym only three times per week and her weight loss averaged only 1.5 pounds per week. Her conclusion was that those extra days at the gym helped her accomplish her goal.

And finally, another great benefit of exercise is that it lifts your mood, a big plus when you are on a controversial eating plan that has many vocal critics.

Finding Time to Exercise

The most common reason people give for not exercising is that they cannot find the time to do it. Nearly all exercise experts agree that it is important to choose a comfortable form of exercise that you can work into your schedule, especially in the beginning. If you have a limited amount of time in which to exercise, strength training (weight lifting) is usually recommended, since it is the best way to add muscle and increase your metabolism in the shortest length of time. But nearly all forms of exercise are beneficial, and you should choose a form that is comfortable and enjoyable for you. You do not need to go to extremes; even if you can add only a short walk a few times a week, you will notice some benefit.

Here are some great tricks and time savers used by seasoned low carbohydrate dieters:

- Betty looks at exercise as being as important to her health as grooming or taking a bath. Most people would never go two to three days without taking a bath or washing their hair. Exercise should be viewed as being just as beneficial.

- When Rosa is returning from an outing with her family in their car, she has them drop her off about a mile away and she walks home. This short walk takes very little time out of her day, yet it returns great rewards.

- Maryanne works in extra exercise at work. First, she parks her car in the farthest parking lot from her job at a large urban hospital and walks to her office. Second, she takes the stairs rather than the elevator to move throughout the building. Since the building has 17 floors, this adds quite a bit of exercise to her day.

- Joseph sets up his laptop computer in front of his treadmill. The only time he allows himself to read his newsgroup messages is when he is on the treadmill.

- Marion does something very similar. She is an avid reader and mixes her love of books with exercise. In the winter, she allows herself to read only when she is on her indoor stationary bicycle. She says she is always surprised at how fast the time goes when she is engrossed in a good book. In warmer weather, she allows herself to listen to books on tape only when she is walking. She says that by combining exercise and books, she not only exercises more, but she reads more too.

- Ruth keeps herself motivated by walking with a neighbor. They both find that this helps them exercise on days they do not feel like it because each has a commitment to the other.

- William tried a similar approach but chose a four-legged partner rather than a neighbor. He went to the local animal shelter, adopted a young dog, and began to walk with her each day. Every morning, the dog is ready and enthusiastic for their daily walk.

- Jerry tells himself that all he must do is put on his shoes and walk for five minutes and he can return home. He says that after five minutes, he is enjoying it so much that he almost always extends the walk for half an hour or more.
- Sherry says she promises herself that she can have a treat if she exercises for at least 30 minutes. She says that by the time she finishes her walk, she feels so much better and so much more motivated to stick to the diet that she no longer wants the treat.

Include the Whole Family

The parents of young children often have a particularly difficult time fitting exercise into their lives. Many find that the trick is to combine their exercise time with their family time and take care of both needs at once. While it may take some effort to get everyone coordinated, it can be done. The first step is to turn off the television. Nearly every family can squeeze at least 30 minutes a day from their schedule by doing this one simple thing. Besides, all those television ads for high carbohydrate products can stimulate carbohydrate cravings and weaken your resistance. Most of us find that the less we see of the doughboy, the better.

For example, Rick is the working father of a preschooler who says he finds it very difficult to add exercise to the list of responsibilities that come along with having a family and a busy career. But he found a solution that allows him at least one hour of walking per week. On Saturday mornings, Rick and his wife and daughter walk to a restaurant near their home that serves breakfast. The walk to the restaurant is a pleasant stroll that consists of mostly down-hill terrain and takes about 25 minutes. Once they arrive,

Rick and his daughter share a big breakfast platter; he eats the low carbohydrate bacon and eggs, and his normal-weighted child eats the pancakes and syrup. Rick says he is motivated not to overeat because the walk back home is all uphill and much more rigorous. If he overeats, he cannot breathe well enough to make it back. It takes the family about 35 minutes to walk back home. Rick's total exercise time adds up to about an hour.

By creatively including the whole family in his Saturday morning hour of exercise, Rick says he gains benefits that last all week. He gets an immediate, large boost in energy that lasts for two to three days. He almost always loses an appreciable amount of weight during the following week. His wife and child also have fun exercising, and their mood improves along with his. And best of all, he finds that he and his family connect emotionally through this family ritual. They actually find the time to talk to one another away from telephones, cell phones, beepers, television, and radios, a benefit they find hard to achieve in their otherwise busy week.

Another way that Rick works exercise into his busy schedule is by taking his daughter to the community indoor pool. He says the trick is to put down his book, get out of his poolside chair, and jump in! Not only does he get great exercise and a boost in metabolism, but wearing his swimming trunks also reminds him of his weight loss goal.

Following are some other great activity ideas that will get you and your family moving:

- *Take a bicycle ride.* Every child loves bicycle rides, and great devices are on the market that will allow even the youngest member of the family to go along.
- *Go on a nature walk.* What child does not like to go on a long exploration? Go along with them, and you may

find that you not only lose weight but regain a bit of your childhood wonder as well.

- *Get involved in your child's sport.* Volunteering to be a coach or referee for your child's sports team can keep you on the run and burning calories while being an active part of your child's life.
- *Go to the park.* Take the children to the park along with another adult, such as your spouse or a neighbor. While the children get great exercise on the playground equipment, you and your companion can take turns walking around the park.
- *Take dance lessons.* Dancing is a great activity for couples that not only burns energy and strengthens muscles, but can also put some zip back into a marriage. Another great thing about dancing is that it is great exercise for people of any age and can be done alone, in couples, or as a family. Square dancing is a family favorite.

When to Add Exercise

Generally, seasoned low carbohydrate dieters do not recommend adding or increasing exercise in the very early stages of the diet. Adding or increasing exercise while your body is withdrawing from its carbohydrate addiction or switching to an alternative fuel source can be overwhelming and counterproductive. Many people have reported a brief decline in their ability to exercise early on, and if you are new to the diet, you should expect this. Even people accustomed to exercise find that their endurance is lessened in the beginning of the diet. You should add or increase exercise only after you feel that your body has adjusted to the diet. This adjustment happens at different times for different people, but it usually takes a couple of weeks, and it may take longer. You will know when you are ready, and you should wait for the right time.

On the other hand, you should not use waiting for your body to fully adjust as an excuse to unnecessarily delay exercise. While you may feel a little more fatigued at first, your body will adjust, and you can gradually increase your exercise level. You should not push yourself too hard, but then again, you should not be afraid to jump in and get started. For example, Ted is a low carbohydrate dieter who was a runner for years. His ability to run weakened noticeably at first. He felt sluggish during the first couple of months of his low carbohydrate diet, but after a while, his endurance came back to him "in a rush." Now he feels he is running better than before.

Exercising in some fashion is important. Once you are ready, approach it gradually. Begin with a mild exercise, such as walking, and gradually build up to a more strenuous one, especially if you have not exercised for a while. Allow yourself some time to build up the endurance, self-confidence, stamina, and general good health that will make you a success in the long run. People who use a "slow but steady" approach and let their bodies guide them find that their bodies adjust and their stamina improves as they go along.

For example, Leonard did not follow the "start slowly" advice and exercised vigorously. As a result, he suffered multiple overuse injuries, and his ability to exercise regularly was inhibited because of them. Worst of all, he did not enjoy it. After a while, he finally heeded the advice and began again. This time, he approached it more gradually. He began walking on a treadmill until his injuries healed. The treadmill improved his stamina and strength, but after a while, he got bored with it. He then started cycling. Not only did he get a great deal of injury-free exercise while riding his bike, he also found that the stamina and strength he had gained during his treadmill workouts allowed him to enjoy it. His enthusiasm caused him to ride a bit too much on his first time out, but his legs were now much stronger and he did not injure himself. He was eventually able to complete a 16-mile ride that included several hills, and he felt great. In retrospect, he concluded that he was simply trying to do too much too soon at first. His advice is to start slowly, increase slowly, and stick with it.

A word of caution: As discussed in Chapter 2, adding or increasing exercise may not immediately show benefits on your scale. In fact, in the short term (the first few days or weeks), exercise may temporarily increase your scale weight. Likewise, you may have a brief period in which you notice a slight increase in size, as the stimulated muscles take up extra blood and fluid and begin to grow. Your body will adjust, however, and the fat loss that was occurring all along will become evident as your size decreases. A body fat analyzer can be very helpful in measuring the shift from fat to muscle during this period of adjustment.

Exercise can increase your need for water beyond the recommendations given earlier in this chapter, especially if you exercise outdoors in warm or hot weather. Consult your physician before beginning an exercise program, especially if you have not been exercising regularly, have a medical condition or illness, or have a great deal of weight to lose.

Shake Things Up

Some people find that after a while on a low carbohydrate diet, their bodies establish a state of equilibrium and their weight loss begins to slow or stops altogether. The current theory is that over time, our bodies make adjustments to our new eating style and begin to establish new ways of managing the metabolic processes that are necessary for daily life. For those of us who have a propensity to gain and maintain extra fat stores, the body adjusts its metabolic outputs based upon its recent history of food intake and energy output. The idea is to shake things up a bit by changing your routine to force your body out of its static state and begin losing weight again. This can be accomplished by changing your exercise routine and your eating routines.

Change Your Exercise Regime

If you have been exercising for a while and your rate of weight loss is slowing or you are stuck in a plateau, you may need to shake things up a bit. Doing a variety of exercises is important to maximize the amount of energy you burn in the long run. The theory is that when the body becomes accustomed to an exercise that uses the same muscle groups repeatedly, the muscles become more fuel-efficient. Less energy is required to perform the exercise than when it was initiated. Therefore, after a while, the muscle does not burn as many calories as it once did. The second reason to vary your exercise routine is to keep your interest up and decrease the chances that you will reduce the amount you exercise or quit out of boredom.

Try something new. For example, if you usually walk, try playing tennis instead. By switching from walking, an exercise that uses mostly the muscles in your legs and buttocks, to tennis, an exercise that also uses the chest, back, and arm muscles, you may be able to give your metabolism a boost.

If you really love a particular exercise and do not want to

switch, try increasing the amount of time you do it. Or change the time of day you do it. For example, if you ordinarily walk for 30 minutes each morning, try walking for 45 minutes or walk in the evening. Or change the way you perform your exercise. For example, if you usually walk at a steady pace, interject brief periods of a more intense, faster pace for a few minutes before returning to your usual pace. If you generally walk on a level surface, such as on a walking track or in a mall, try walking a nature trail that has some hills.

Change Your Eating Habits

You can also shake things up by changing your eating habits. Many dieters find that over time, they settle into a routine and eat only a few basic foods over and over again. Eating the same foods at the same time of day over a long period of time may cause your body to also become more efficient at digesting these foods.

As discussed in Chapter 3, decreasing or increasing their calorie, carbohydrate, or protein intake has produced results for many reduced carbohydrate dieters. Karen tried shaking things up by dramatically increasing her overall intake for one day. She tracked her intake using a nutrition counter, then increased her intake to a level well above her usual. She says she saw immediate results in that her weight loss once again resumed.

Another tactic is to change the time of day you eat. Breakfast is the meal that generates the most discussion among dieters. Specifically, the discussion centers on the question of whether or not it is advisable to skip breakfast. One school of thought is that skipping breakfast is very detrimental to metabolism. Others report that they are not hungry first thing in the morning and, therefore, feel that eating breakfast is not necessary. Both camps have supporters who cite their experience as evidence for their approach. Jose says that he and his wife were able to speed their weight loss simply by eating their breakfast after ten o'clock (when they took a brisk walk) rather than at their usual eight o'clock (before their walk). Their theory is that the delay in eating breakfast allows their bodies more time to burn fat before they provide food to be used as fuel. They claim that this simple action made a big difference for them, even though their overall intake of food has remained the same.

Others report that eating breakfast again after years of skipping it had a positive effect on them. Jennifer says that after eating breakfast, especially a protein-rich breakfast, she was able to control her hunger much better throughout the remainder of the day. She says that if she does not eat in the morning, her weight loss stalls. Bianca agrees with the importance of eating breakfast. She also says she does not lose weight if she eats too late in the day, especially if she eats immediately before bedtime.

Another successful technique frequently used by low carbohydrate dieters is to eat six mini-meals throughout the day rather than three larger, traditional meals. The theory is that we will keep our insulin levels more stable if we spread our carbohydrate intake out over several hours rather than ingesting it in one sitting. For example, eating six small meals of 8 grams of carbohydrate each, for a total of 48 grams of carbohydrate per day, will cause less insulin to be released, and therefore more weight to be lost, than eating all 48 grams of carbohydrate in one sitting. The proponents of this theory state that eating all 48 grams of carbohydrate at one time risks an insulin spike that will be followed by a blood sugar dip that will set off carbohydrate cravings and unnecessary hunger. (It is important to note that the authors of *The Carbohydrate Addict's Diet* do not agree with this advice.)

You may also need to change what you eat. You can shake things up by expanding your selection of foods by investing in one of the many low carbohydrate cookbooks currently available. Many of the reduced carbohydrate Internet sites also have sections where participants post their favorite low carbohydrate recipes. While some of these may not be fully kitchen-tested for quality and taste, they are usually free and can be a great foundation for developing your own creations. Joan says that she was able to greatly expand the variety in her meals by surfing the recipe sections of the reduced carbohydrate message boards. Preparing great reduced carbohydrate meals helps her remember that there is variety and enjoyment in reduced carbohydrate eating. She especially enjoys adding sauces for meat back to her menus. By expanding her recipe assortment, she says she became much less susceptible to the carbohydrate cravings that sprang from food boredom. (For a list of reduced carbohydrate cookbooks and Internet recipe sites, see Chapter 6.)

Change Your Diet Plan

Some dieters have taken a suggestion from Dr. Atkins to go off the diet for one to three days or so to accelerate their rate of weight loss. This is a technique that Dr. Atkins calls a reversal diet in his book *Dr. Atkins' New Diet Revolution*. The idea is that by going on another diet for a short period and then returning to low carbohydrate dieting, you should be able to recapture the rapid weight loss that you experienced early in the diet. He cautions that going off the low carbohydrate diet should not be used as an excuse to binge; you must go onto another diet in which calories are restricted. While it is acceptable to return to eating carbohydrate during this short break, you should continue to avoid simple sugars. Most of your carbohydrate intake should continue to be in the form of complex carbohydrate, such as from vegetables. You should not chew through a bag of cookies. This technique worked very well for Mick. He says he broke a plateau by shocking his system by going off his diet for a few days. He immediately followed these few days of off-plan eating with a return to the initial (lowest carbohydrate) stage of his plan.

While some people have taken Dr. Atkins' suggestion and found that it did indeed speed their weight loss, others report that they do not like the brief weight gain, water retention, and other uncomfortable symptoms that accompany it. Still others report that even though the length of time they were off the diet was brief, they found themselves struggling to break their carbohydrate addiction again once they returned to their reduced carbohydrate diet.

Trey tells of his trip down a "slippery slope" that led him back to his carbohydrate addiction. After months of faithful low carbohydrate dieting, he found he was stuck in a long plateau. So he took a little vacation from his diet for about two days. When he returned to low carbohydrate eating, he experienced one of his best weeks of weight loss. But as with all addictions, now that he had indulged in carbohydrate again, he found himself on a slippery slope. About two weeks later, he took another little vacation with the same results—a great weight loss when he returned. However, he found that it was now extremely hard for him to stop eating carbohydrate. His carbohydrate addiction had returned to haunt him.

Trey's time between vacations from low carbohydrate eating became shorter and shorter, while the time he spent off the plan became longer and longer. Before he knew it, he had regained several pounds. He was able to break his addiction to carbohydrate and get back on track once again, but not until after he returned to the basics of his chosen plan and started all over. The lesson he learned was that he would have to follow his diet consistently to control his carbohydrate addiction.

Take Nutritional Supplements

As is the case with any diet, it is important to take a wide variety of vitamins, minerals, and other nutrients each day. Many reduced carbohydrate diet book authors strongly believe that vitamin and mineral deficiencies cripple the body's ability to properly perform biological functions that are critical for weight loss. They assert that weight loss stalls without these important supplements. Many seasoned dieters and many nutritional experts agree that taking adequate vitamins reduces the food cravings that may result from vitamin and mineral deficiencies and, therefore, prevents overeating. The risk is that these cravings will lead to increased carbohydrate and calorie intake, which, in turn, will slow weight loss and cause plateaus.

While nearly everyone, seasoned dieters and experts alike, agrees that adding vitamins and minerals to our diet is important, the question becomes which ones to include and which ones to exclude. This is truly an example of when "the devil dwells in the detail." The topic of which supplements enhance metabolism and increase weight loss and which ones are a waste of money always generates lively discussions among reduced carbohydrate dieters. The topic is often complex and can be confusing because the number of supplements discussed is quite large. The matter is further complicated by the fact that Internet newsgroups are peppered with participants trying to market nutritional supplements to other participants. (The message board sponsors and participants refer to these messages as "spam." They strongly discourage this practice, but it occurs nonetheless. It is often disguised as friendly advice.)

Not only should we be wary of the motivations of people giving testimonials, but we should also be skeptical of claims that have not been tested by traditional research. The fact that many claims are untested allows sellers a great deal of latitude in promoting their products. Every few weeks, news of a promising new supplement that claims to speed weight loss bursts onto the scene. Over time, the false promise fades as the reduced carbohydrate dieters who try them are disappointed. However, not all nutritional supplements are failures.

Recommended Supplements

Some of the reduced carbohydrate diet book authors strongly believe that certain vitamins, minerals, and other nutritional supplements have a profound effect on the success of a reduced carbohydrate diet. In fact, more than one of them have devoted whole chapters of their diet books to the subject, while a couple of them wrote separate books on the topic. Of the books discussed in Chapter 1, four of them—*Dr. Atkins' New Diet Revolution, Protein Power, The Schwarzbein Principle,* and *Thin for Good*— contain detailed recommendations regarding nutritional supplementation. In these four books, over 80 nutrients are mentioned.

Discussing all of these nutrients is well beyond the scope of this book. In the interest of brevity, we will discuss just the nutrients that are mentioned in all four books. If you are interested in more information about nutritional supplements, review the four diet books. The nutrients recommended in all four books are:

- *Chromium.* Of all the supplements mentioned by the reduced carbohydrate diet book authors, chromium is the most frequently discussed and recommended. Chromium is believed to be important in facilitating the action of insulin at the receptor sites. It is believed to promote muscle building, increase fat breakdown, and decrease cholesterol levels. Chromium deficiency is believed to be a major cause of carbohydrate cravings and a major contributor to the development of insulin resistance.

- *Essential fatty acids (EFAs).* The essential fatty acids are fatty acids that cannot be manufactured by the body and therefore must be obtained from the diet. Many nutritionists recommend taking essential fatty acid supplements because the EFAs are essential for life. The EFAs specifically recommended are omega-3s, omega-6s, and linoleic acid.

- *B-complex vitamins.* The B-complex vitamins mentioned in the four diet books are biotin, niacin (vitamin B_3), cyanocobalamin (vitamin B_{12}), pyridoxine (vitamin B_6), riboflavin (vitamin B_2), and thiamine (vitamin B_1). For these B vitamins to be fully effective, folic acid should also be taken. The B vitamins are believed to have a positive effect on energy, mood, carbohydrate metabolism, blood sugar stabilization, protein metabolism, serotonin production, eye function, brain function, nervous system function, and blood cell formation.

- *Vitamin C (ascorbic acid).* Vitamin C is believed to

have a wide range of benefits, not the least of which is
to help protect against heart disease.

* *Carnitine.* The general consensus among reduced carbohydrate dieters is that carnitine is very helpful in
weight loss. Carnitine, also referred to as L-carnitine,
is believed to be important in the transport of fats and
some vitamins in the body. It is also credited for promoting healthy heart function. A deficiency of carnitine is believed to contribute to difficulty in losing
body fat. Dr. Atkins states that a lack of carnitine is a
contributing factor for overweight people who are unable to get into ketosis.

Potassium

Potassium deserves special mention because it is one of
the more important minerals and should be taken daily
while on a reduced carbohydrate diet, especially by people
who are on ketogenic diets. Potassium has a potent effect
on heart rhythm and other critical body functions, especially the functioning of the nerves and muscles. Potassium also plays a role in carbohydrate metabolism. Low
potassium levels, known medically as hypokalemia (with
hypo meaning "too low," *kal* referring to potassium, and
emia meaning "in the blood") can develop when potassium
is flushed from the body along with the water that is released with diuresis. A low potassium level can lead to serious problems, especially in people who have certain
medical conditions. Because potassium affects the functioning of the heart, nerves, and muscles, the symptoms of
low potassium are evident in these organs and tissues.
Symptoms of hypokalemia are irregular heartbeat, tingling
in the hands and feet, light-headedness, muscle aches,

muscle fatigue, and depression. The most common complaints are muscle fatigue and cramping. The muscle fatigue tends to be generalized and affects all the muscles, while the muscle cramps tend to occur deep in the major muscle groups, such as the legs (they can be quite painful).

Many low carbohydrate dieters find they must continually replace potassium through supplements. Potassium is available over the counter in 99-milligram tablets. It is also the main ingredient in many "light salt" and "no salt" products, which tend to be considerably cheaper than potassium supplements. It also occurs naturally in many foods.

A word of caution: While taking potassium every day is very important, you should consult your physician to determine how much potassium supplementation is appropriate for you, especially if you have a medical condition. Too much potassium can also lead to serious problems. It can have strong interactions with prescription and over-the-counter medications as well. There is no recommended daily allowance for potassium, and the amount of supplementation you require depends upon several factors that you should discuss with your physician.

Designer Supplements

Dr. Atkins believes so strongly in the benefits of adequate nutritional supplementation that he has developed a line of products he describes as targeted nutrition. These supplements, known as the Vita-Nutrient Supplements, are specifically designed for low carbohydrate dieters. Their purpose is to boost energy, boost metabolism, squelch carbohydrate cravings, and protect against disease. This brand of supplements is commonly recommended to people who are chronically slow losers, are stuck in plateaus, or have significant carbohydrate cravings. Some people have found success with them and have reported that the benefits were well worth the expense.

Mark is now a supporter of designer supplements. He says he was put off initially by their cost and opted instead for what he called "drugstore vitamins" plus extra potassium. When he developed a long plateau, he began to research the topic in detail. One of the books he read (a book not written by Dr. Atkins) convinced him that improper vitamin supplementation is indeed a major cause of decreased metabolism and plateaus. He purchased Dr. Atkins' supplements and broke through his plateau in less than a week.

Laela also discounted the benefits of designer supplements in the first year of her low carbohydrate diet. While she was successful at losing weight, she lost it slowly, as she struggled with carbohydrate cravings. After trying Dr. Atkins' supplements for a month, she reported her appetite was down, her energy level was up, and her weight loss was easier and quicker.

Whether you invest in supplements that are designed for low carbohydrate dieters or not, at a minimum you should take a high-quality, comprehensive multivitamin each day.

A word of caution: While certain nutritional supplements are believed to be beneficial for reduced carbohydrate dieters, you should not take any of them without consulting your physician first, especially if you have a medical condition or are taking a prescription drug. Some supplements can have a powerful, pronounced effect on body functions and can interact with other drugs, including over-the-counter and prescription medications. Professional advice is always a necessary step in determining the right mixture of nutritional supplements.

Keep It Simple

Some low carbohydrate dieters recommend a plateau-breaking practice featuring foods that are natural, simply prepared, and very low in carbohydrate. This method is known as the Keep It Simple, Sweetheart method (known as KISS for short), and it need be practiced for just a few days.

Recommended foods in the KISS method include unprocessed meats cooked in oil, fresh, low carbohydrate vegetables, and a lot of water. Some dieters also add a few other oils such as mayonnaise, but for the most part restrict themselves to meats and low carbohydrate vegetables. The idea is to remove all of the agents that could be causing the plateau in an effort to break it.

Meat Fast

One extreme technique for breaking plateaus that is the subject of frequent debates among low carbohydrate dieters is the meat fast. In the meat fast, total carbohydrate intake is kept as close as possible to 0 grams for one to two days by eating only meat, the oil necessary to prepare it, and water. Meat is eaten as the only food for two reasons. First, it provides the body with enough protein to minimize the breakdown of muscle and other lean body tissues. Second, it is one of the few protein-based foods that are truly carbohydrate-free. (Processed meat products contain small amounts of carbohydrate, so they are not included in the meat fast.)

Many dieters who have tried the meat fast report it produced a quick weight loss, sometimes of as much as several pounds. They say this rapid loss is similar to what they experienced in the first couple of weeks on their diets.

Further, they claim that once their plateaus were broken, their weight loss continued even after they returned to their normal reduced carbohydrate diets.

Carly is a low carbohydrate dieter who tried the meat fast. In the first year of her diet, she experienced two major stalls. The first, about four months into the diet, lasted for about six weeks. She chose to do the meat fast for one day while increasing the amount of water she drank. The next morning, she found she had lost a significant amount of weight. Although she returned to her usual low carbohydrate diet the next day, her weight loss continued. Her second plateau occurred approximately nine months into her diet and lasted for about seven weeks. Once again, she tried the meat fast for one day, and she had the same great results. Her plateau ended and her weight loss continued after she returned to eating her previous level of carbohydrate.

However, some people who have tried this technique report it is very bland and boring and can set off carbohydrate binges. Reanna's goal was to meat fast for two days. By the second day, she said, she was so bored and restless that carbohydrate cravings were beginning to mount. By the evening of the second day, her carbohydrate cravings were much stronger than ever before. This strong craving set her off eating popcorn at first. Then, she says, she "lost her mind" and began cutting a swath through her kitchen looking for sugar. When it was over, she had devoured a box of chocolates. She says that when she awoke the next morning, she felt terrible and was not sure what had happened. Her low carbohydrate peers told her it sounded like a classic flare-up of carbohydrate addiction precipitating a binge. Reanna says she will not try the meat fast again.

Many people are very concerned about the meat fast and discourage others from using it. While nearly everyone agrees that eating only meat for a very short period of one to two days, and doing it infrequently, is not likely to cause any significant harm, many people feel the practice is open to abuse and overuse. They warn that overdoing it can leave you prone to nutritional deficiencies, which are a major cause of the carbohydrate cravings and metabolic disturbances that can lead to weight gain.

They also warn that because the protein and fat in meat cause a great deal of satiety, you can be prone to undereating. Taking in too few calories is a well-known cause of slowed metabolism. Therefore, overuse of the meat fast can lead to an even more difficult stall later.

Perhaps the most compelling argument against the meat fast is the contention that it can trigger eating disorders in those who are prone to them. Many people feel the meat fast is an extreme form of dieting. They object that it is contrary to the philosophy that reduced carbohydrate dieting is a healthy way of living and not a temporary fix to a long-term problem. For many reduced carbohydrate dieters, the potential of using the meat fast as a way to lose a great deal of weight quickly is in direct opposition to the healthy principles of the reduced carbohydrate way of life.

Despite the fact that the wisdom of the meat fast is regularly questioned and debated among reduced carbohydrate dieters, and virtually none of the reduced carbohydrate diet book authors mention it in their books, it has gained momentum. If you choose to use the meat fast technique, you should do so infrequently. You should do it only after you have been stuck in a plateau and have lost no weight or inches for several weeks. You should use it only after you have ruled out all the causes of stalls and plateaus discussed in Chapter 3 and have applied all other techniques to break them discussed in this chapter. The length of the meat fast should also be short, only one or two days at a time. Be sure to take adequate nutritional supplements during it. Do not use the technique simply to speed weight loss. Be sure to drink a great deal of water with it. And if you have a history of eating disorders, approach the technique with a great deal of caution.

Develop Strategies to Control Binges

Let's face it. Falling off the wagon is a natural part of dieting, and reduced carbohydrate dieting is no exception. We all suffer from carbohydrate cravings and subsequent binges, especially early in the diet. Many seasoned dieters say that binges are much less common on reduced carbohydrate diets than on low fat diets, but they occur nonetheless. The most common time for binges is early in the diet; most people report that binges become less and less frequent the more accustomed they become to the reduced carbohydrate lifestyle.

For successful dieters, the most effective binge control strategy has three essential components. First, it includes methods for preventing binges. Second, it includes methods to limit binges once they begin. And lastly, it includes methods for recovering from binges.

Preventing Binges

Without a doubt, the best strategy for dealing with carbohydrate binges is to prevent them from occurring in the first place. Many of us have a variety of strategies for preventing binges, and while many of these strategies have already been discussed, they are worth repeating briefly here. In the spirit of "the best defense is a good offense," we should first strive to prevent the very conditions that lead to binges. Following are the techniques widely believed to be the best ways to do so:

- *Take vitamins regularly*. Many experts believe that nutritional deficiencies are one of the primary reasons strong urges to eat strike dieters. Proponents of this theory believe that our bodies send out crude signals to eat when vital nutrients are lacking. It would be great if our bodies would send out specific signals, such as, "Excuse me, I need more B_{12} please," but unfortunately, the signal comes across as a strong craving instead. So, to prevent binges caused by nutritional deficiencies, take a high-quality, broad-spectrum multi-vitamin-and-mineral supplement each day, along with extra potassium. Many seasoned dieters and diet experts alike also recommend taking L-carnitine, a nutrient widely believed to decrease carbohydrate cravings.
- *Eat adequate protein*. Protein deprivation can be a strong trigger for binge eating. This is especially true for people who are adding muscle through new or increased exercise. If you are experiencing strong urges to binge, especially in the evening, you may need to examine your daily protein intake to ensure you are getting enough.
- *Eat frequent mini-meals*. Going too long between meals can allow your hunger to go unchecked and your blood sugar levels to drop too low. Consider eating smaller, more frequent meals to maintain control over your hunger and to stabilize your blood sugar levels. (Note that the authors of *The Carbohydrate Addict's Diet* do not agree with this advice, as they recommend eating all carbohydrate at one meal.)
- *Drink plenty of fluids*. Some people mistake thirst sig-

nals for hunger signals. If you are seriously dehydrated and misinterpret the thirst signal as hunger, it can lead to a binge.

- *Get plenty of sleep.* Fatigue can be a major trigger for overeating and bingeing for all dieters. First of all, when we are tired, our resistance to any temptation is down. But more important, many people commonly misinterpret their need for rest as a need for food. It is as though they think eating more food will give them the energy they are missing from lack of sleep.

- *Identify and avoid your triggers.* Over time, you will be able to identify which foods trigger binges for you. Commonly cited food triggers are products containing artificial sweeteners, such as diet soft drinks, drink mixes, candy, gum, gelatins, puddings, and syrups; caffeine; wine and other spirits; whipped cream; chocolate; nuts; and "sugar-free" snacks. Other common triggers are stress and depression.

Limiting Binges

Since urges to binge are certain to strike despite the best-laid plans to prevent them, you should develop methods to limit their severity once they begin. The sooner you realize that a binge is coming on and the earlier you employ your strategy, the better. At first, this can be hard to do, as new low carbohydrate dieters are often taken by surprise by a binge. However, over time, you will learn your body's responses to reduced carbohydrate dieting, and you will be able to recognize the signs of an oncoming binge earlier and earlier. The following methods are frequently used by dieters as binge-stoppers. If possible, employ these methods before the binge gets fully underway. However, if you are a victim of a spontaneous ambush of strong cravings, try to employ them as soon as possible. Your goal will then be to interrupt or shorten the duration of the binge.

- *De-stress yourself.* Many people find success using relaxation techniques when they are in the grips of a strong urge to splurge brought on by stress. For example, when Sherry recognizes an approaching binge related to stress, she promises herself she can have anything she wishes after a 30-minute walk. By the time she returns from her walk, she is relaxed, her appetite is suppressed, and she rarely wants the food she was craving so badly before.
- *Drink water.* If your urge to binge is caused by dehydration, drinking water can quickly limit the severity of the binge. The best method is to drink 16 ounces of water about 20 minutes before you indulge in the binge. However, if you find yourself halfway through a bag of chips before you realize you are really thirsty, not hungry, you should still pause and drink two glasses of water to try to interrupt the binge. Drinking water will squelch the thirst that caused the binge in the first place, and it will also make your stomach feel fuller.
- *Take a break.* If possible, take a 30-minute nap. This can be an amazingly successful strategy, especially if your urges are brought on by fatigue or stress. If a nap is not possible, as it often is not, at least try to find a quiet place to rest and meditate. Even the most hectic and stressful workplaces have some alcove in which you can find seclusion for a few minutes, such as the bathroom.
- *Eat protein and fiber.* If your binge was precipitated by hunger because you waited too long between

meals, eat foods that are high in protein and fiber until your hunger is in check. Protein and high fiber foods have the advantage of raising the blood sugar slowly and evenly. Therefore, the risk of causing a large release of insulin is lessened.

- *Have alternatives on hand.* Having protein and high fiber foods readily available to ward off binges requires planning ahead so they are on hand when the urge strikes. Having your favorite low carbohydrate treat handy may also do the trick.

- *Limit the time frame.* Some reduced carbohydrate dieters adopt the recommendations of the Hellers in *The Carbohydrate Addict's Diet* and limit their binge to 60 minutes. If possible, follow the rest of the Hellers' advice and eat one-third protein, one-third low carbohydrate vegetables, and one-third carbohydrate.

- *Use your head.* Some people use intellectual reason as a method to limit a binge. The best rule to remember is: The more carbohydrate you eat, the more carbohydrate your body must burn through before it can return to burning your body fat. In other words, a little indiscretion is no reason to indulge further. Using the excuse, "Oh well, since I have already blown it by having this piece of candy, I may as well have a piece of cake and some ice cream, too," is a sure path to extending the damage of a binge. Keep in mind that a little carbohydrate will stop your weight loss for a few hours, but a full-blown binge can stop it for much longer—or even worse, cause weight gain.

Recovering From Binges

Oh . . . the morning after. It hurts. Literally. Physically, you are bloated because the carbohydrate you ate caused your body to hold large amounts of water. Psychologically, you feel like a failure. Mentally, your brain is a fog. You have gas, and you probably have a lot of it. Seasoned low carbohydrate dieters say that this is the critical time that separates the successful dieters from the ones who do not make it. The ones who quit say, "I knew this diet would not work. It is impossible to maintain. The critics were right." The ones who go on to lose more weight pick themselves up, get over it, and get right back on track. Here are several methods that will help you be one of the ones who make it:

- *Do not weigh yourself for 48 hours.* You already know how bad the damage is—you can feel it. Your scale weight the morning after will only exaggerate your perception of the damage. If you ate a large amount of carbohydrate, especially if it was simple, refined carbohydrate, you gained a lot of water weight. This will be magnified if you were in ketosis before the binge and now you are not. Your scale weight will reflect all the water you gained and will not tell you how much fat you gained. If you are lucky, all of your weight gain will be made up of water and none of body fat, but you will not be able to ascertain this for about 48 hours after your return to low carbohydrate eating. Looking at the scale the morning after will not serve any purpose other than deepening your regret.

- *Get back on track.* This is the best advice by far. Start right away with the basics of your food plan. If your plan recommends an introduction stage, repeat it. By jumping right back on the wagon, you minimize the effects of the binge. Do not be tempted to starve yourself the following day in an effort to reverse the damage of the binge. This could set you off on a roller coaster of low blood sugar followed by another binge.

• *Forgive yourself.* The only thing that binges prove is that we are not perfect. Unless you are under the age of ten, you should already know that. Get over it and move on. We all make mistakes. Use what you have learned to increase your chances of success in the future. The difference between people who are successful and those who fail is not that the successful never stumble and fall—they simply pick themselves up and start over.

Ephedrine and ECA Stacking

Some people who are chronically slow losers, are stuck in a long plateau, or simply want to speed their rate of weight loss turn to the herb ephedrine for help. Ephedrine is a nerve stimulant that has a well-known energizing effect. In essence, it is a naturally occurring stimulant or "speed." For weight loss purposes, ephedrine is classified as a nutritional supplement, and it is sold in health food stores, health food sections of stores, and little booths at shopping malls. It has many names, including ephedra, *Ephedra sinica,* and ma huang (its Chinese name). Ephedrine is marketed as an energy-booster, metabolism-booster, and thermogenic or fat-burning supplement. (Note that ephedrine is not pseudoephedrine.)

Using ephedrine for weight loss is very controversial. While many people report that ephedrine sped up their weight loss, others warn that its risks far outweigh its benefits. Its boosting effect has been directly linked with heartbeat irregularities, and the FDA has issued warnings regarding its use since at least 1994. Among its serious side effects are dizziness, severe headache, rapid heartbeat, irregular heartbeat, chest pain, shortness of breath, hypertension, nausea, loss of consciousness, nervousness, anxiety, and significant changes in behavior. The FDA warns that "taking more than the recommended dose may result in heart attack, stroke, seizure, and/or death." Several states have banned the sale of ephedrine after deaths were directly linked to its use.

The manufacturers of products containing ephedrine counter the FDA's criticism by stating that the deaths resulted from taking larger doses of ephedrine than recommended. Therefore, the labels on most ephedrine products strongly warn against exceeding the recommended dosage. Overdoses typically occur when users increase their dosage after building up a tolerance to the "speedy" side effects. They mistakenly believe that because the side effects are no longer as pronounced, the drug now has a lesser effect on their bodies. In fact, while a few of the side effects may subside as a user becomes accustomed to the herb, the effects on the heart and other organs, including the thermogenic effect, remain the same. For this reason, doses over the recommended amounts should never be taken.

Product labels warn that ephedrine should not be used if you have, or have a family history of, heart disease, thyroid disease, diabetes, high blood pressure, recurrent headaches, depression, psychiatric conditions, glaucoma, difficulty urinating, prostate enlargement, or seizure disorder.

A practice known as ECA stacking is even more controversial than using ephedrine alone. ECA stacking is the combining of other substances with ephedrine to boost the effect of ephedrine even further. "ECA" stands for the three ingredients that are "stacked": Ephedrine, Caffeine, and Aspirin. Stacking is even more strongly discouraged by the FDA than the use of ephedrine alone, but it is regularly practiced nonetheless, especially among dieters interested in bodybuilding.

Another compelling argument against using ephedrine and other "boosting" supplements is that they tend to have a negative impact on our ability to sleep. As discussed in Chapter 3, reduced sleep quality often leads to daytime fatigue, which in turn leads to increased carbohydrate cravings and decreased resistance to them. In this way, taking ephedrine often backfires for those using it to boost weight loss. To combat the negative side effects such as sleep disturbances, some people take ephedrine or ECA stacks for a few days and then skip them for a few days—a practice known as cycling.

Lisa and her friends are good examples of how ephedrine can have varied effects. Lisa began taking a product containing ephedrine because of its promise to boost her metabolism and energy. She found that it gave her just the right amount of "lift," and it also gave her back some of the energy she had had in her youth. She also says that her weight loss seemed easier. However, when her friend tried the same product, she had a very negative experience. Her friend took the recommended dose before work one morning and by mid-morning was very ill. She was jittery and nauseated and her heart was beating wildly. She had to leave work for the remainder of the day.

If you are considering using ephedrine or ECA stacking, you should do some thorough homework before taking it. You should learn the potential effects of all three of the ingredients. You should not take ephedrine or proceed with stacking without consulting your physician *first,* especially if you are under care for a medical condition. All three of the stacking ingredients, especially ephedrine, can have strong effects on your body and can interact negatively with other over-the-counter and prescription drugs. For example, ephedrine is frequently included as an ingredient in over-the-counter breathing medications, and taking both products together can lead to an overdose.

Even with your physician's approval, you should start with small doses. Some people who are sensitive to ephedrine experience substantial nervousness and heartbeat irregularities with their first dose. Experienced users often recommend taking 25 percent of the full dose and certainly no more than half of the full dose for the first few days. By taking a small dose in the beginning and gradually "ramping up" to a full dose over a period of a few days or weeks, you can learn how ephedrine affects you. Proponents say that the dose should be low enough to provide energy without causing hyperactivity or producing a "crash" when it wears off. Increase the dose gradually as the "jittery" side effects subside. Never exceed the maximum dose.

If you are considering ECA stacking, make sure you purchase an ephedrine product that is not already stacked—in other words, it should not already have caffeine and aspirin in it. Purchase the ingredients separately at first. Add the caffeine and aspirin gradually and only after you have determined that you can tolerate the ephedrine.

Heed the warning labels on all the products. Do not take more than the maximum amount specified per dose or per day. Do not take the products for prolonged periods of time. Check all your medications, especially medications for asthma or other breathing problems, for the presence of ephedrine. If you experience any side effects, immediately stop taking it. If you have serious side effects such as heartbeat irregularity, loss of consciousness, or extreme anxiety, seek immediate medical attention.

Get a Medical Checkup

If you are losing weight very slowly or are stuck in a long plateau, get a medical checkup if you have not done so recently. There are many reasons for slow weight loss, and only a trained professional can help you identify some of them. While you should educate yourself using the wealth of information available on reduced carbohydrate dieting, the best thing you can do is develop a good working relationship with a supportive physician.

Some people are reluctant to tell their physicians they are on reduced carbohydrate diets for fear the physician will not approve and will try to talk them out of it. Many people are pleasantly surprised when their physicians actually support their decision. Luckily, finding a supportive doctor is not as difficult as it was just a few short years ago. Macey, who was on a low carbohydrate diet for several months, says she was stunned to overhear her physician actually recommend a reduced carbohydrate diet to another patient.

If your physician is not willing to support your choice of reduced carbohydrate dieting, you always have the option of finding one who does. Reduced carbohydrate Internet groups are a great resource for referrals to supportive physicians. In fact, several physicians participate in the newsgroups to become more familiar with the diet. For example, Diedre asked for a referral to a supportive physician in her city and received three names in less than a day.

There are also physician referral databases on the Internet and at nearly every hospital. These hotlines can be a great source of information about the physicians in your community. If these databases do not have a list of supportive reduced carbohydrate physicians, get a list of physicians who practice weight management (known as bariatric medicine) or endocrinology, and call their offices and ask. It may take a bit of work, but finding a supportive, experienced physician is worth the time and effort.

If All Else Fails, Don't Give Up

If you have tried all the strategies in this book and find that you are still losing weight slowly or stuck in a plateau, hang in there. Above all, *do not give up!* Most periods of slow weight loss are self-correcting if given enough time. Your body may simply need time to adjust to the demands you are placing on it, especially if you are stuck at a new low weight.

Many people find that it is uplifting to occasionally remind themselves of all the benefits of reduced carbohydrate dieting when the scale is moving slowly. They keep a motivational log that lists these benefits and pull it out when they become frustrated. A few examples of the benefits that are frequently mentioned by reduced carbohydrate dieters are:

- *Reduced weight.* Many people report that reviewing how much weight they have already lost, rather than focusing on how much they have yet to lose, is very motivating for them. The weight may not be coming off as quickly as they would like, but they are making progress. For many people, reduced carbohydrate dieting is the only diet that has worked, and it reversed a long-term trend of gaining weight. Leaving the diet would mean regaining the weight lost thus far.

- *Reduced fat.* Almost everyone reports that their clothes fit better and, as a result, their self-image has improved. Some have even noticed that their body mechanics have changed and they have become more flexible. One woman commented that not only could she tie her shoes with ease now, she no longer makes that irritating grunting noise when she bends over.

- *Increased control.* Many people gain greater control over their eating habits. Severe hunger, serious carbohydrate cravings, and binge eating all but disappear for many of them. This brings a great deal of psychological comfort, but overall self-control also seems to increase. Betty says this is her favorite reward from reduced carbohydrate dieting. After years of feeling as though she were battling her body, she says she now feels as though she has some control over it.

- *Decreased appetite.* Many people list decreased appetite as one of the greatest benefits of reduced carbohydrate eating. Their appetite is down in part because of the increased satiety that comes from eating protein and fat. People in ketosis report that their appetite is even easier to control. Not thinking of food every minute frees them up to do other things. It is not uncommon for people to comment that they did not realize how much of their time had been taken up with food preparation and eating until they became reduced carbohydrate dieters.

- *Stabilized blood sugar.* People who had blood sugar problems report that their blood sugar levels have become much more stable. This includes both diabetics, who suffer from elevated blood sugar levels, and hypoglycemics, who suffer from low blood sugar. Norma is a diabetic who found that low carbohydrate dieting helps her control her blood sugar. When she first tried low carbohydrate dieting, she found she was much more able to control her glucose levels and required only oral medication. In addition, she lost some weight and felt better. However, her nutritionist warned her against low carbohydrate eating, so Norma gave it up and returned to her previous lifestyle of eating carbohydrate. She ended up on insulin, gained 20 pounds, and found herself continually battling high blood glucose readings. When she became fed up, she returned to low carbohydrate eating and now is again able to control her blood sugar using only oral medication. She's lost 15 of the 20 pounds she gained during her break from low carbohydrate dieting and says she feels good again.

- *Improved energy and mood.* Without the peaks and valleys associated with eating carbohydrate, many people find their energy levels and moods consistently better. Patricia said that even if she never loses another pound, she is firmly committed to the reduced carbohydrate lifestyle because of her improved energy level. She reports that for ten years, she had a major energy slump in the mid-afternoon—around two o'clock or three o'clock every day. Some days it was so serious that she had to take a nap to get through the remainder of the afternoon. Since she has been restricting her carbohydrate intake, her energy slump has disappeared along with the need to take daily naps, and her energy level has increased overall.

- *Decreased cholesterol levels.* Many people have reported that their total cholesterol levels have dropped and that their ratio of good cholesterol to bad cholesterol has improved. Ravina battled high cholesterol for about two years before she tried reduced carbohydrate dieting. Even with prescription medication, her triglycerides ranged between 400 and 900, her low density lipoprotein (LDL or bad cholesterol) was close to 300, while her high density lipoprotein (HDL or good cholesterol) was a mere 12. After she tried a low carbohydrate diet for eight weeks and quit smoking, her laboratory tests revealed that her triglycerides were only 116, her LDL had fallen to 131, and her HDL had risen to 42.

- *Decreased water retention.* By limiting their carbohydrate intake, many people find they retain much less water than they did when they ate more carbohydrate. Women find their premenstrual bloating much improved.

- *Decreased hypertension.* Some people report that their hypertension improved as their bodies released the water associated with carbohydrate intake. Andrew, for example, found that his blood pressure dropped to normal levels after three months of low carbohydrate dieting.

- *Reduced migraines.* Migraine sufferers often report they were pleasantly surprised to find that low carbohydrate dieting decreased both the severity and the frequency of their migraines. Andrea says she suffered with migraines for years. The pain regularly interfered with her life, including her relationships, schoolwork, job, and sleep. She tried several recommendations over the years, but had limited success, and her migraines continued nearly on a weekly basis. Many were severe, and she was a regular visitor to emergency rooms for treatment. After starting a low carbohydrate diet, she was astounded that she did not have a single full-blown migraine in nearly two months—a record for her. The few headaches she did experience were more easily treatable and resolved quickly.

- *Improved sleep.* The spouses of low carbohydrate dieters love this benefit. Many people report that their snoring dramatically decreased or stopped altogether. This benefit is widely believed to be directly related to decreasing weight, but some people report they saw an improvement in their snoring even before they lost substantial amounts. Darma says her husband sought treatment for severe snoring and apnea for years. After he went on the low carbohydrate diet, he lost 46 pounds and stopped snoring altogether. Now she reports she loses sleep because he sleeps so quietly that she feels compelled to check him occasionally to be sure he is still breathing!

- *Improved skin, hair, and nails.* As they increased the amount of protein and fat in their diets, many people found that moisture and strength returned to their skin, hair, and nails. This seems to be especially true for people who spent a long time on low fat diets. Myra says that her skin has never been better than in the two years since she began her low carbohydrate lifestyle. She says she consistently gets compliments about her great complexion. One of her parents' neighbors who had not seen her for about eight months repeatedly complimented her on how wonderful her skin looked. Myra says this has given her something to be proud of while waiting to reach her weight loss goal.

- *Decreased gastrointestinal distress.* Many people report that several gastrointestinal problems that plagued them in the past, such as gastric reflux, lactose intolerance, irritable bowel syndrome, colitis, and excess gas, have greatly improved or disappeared altogether. Geneva and George are two low carbohydrate dieters who were once long-term users of multiple prescription medications for indigestion and heartburn. George says he consulted his physician after his heartburn disappeared in the first three months of his low carbohydrate diet. With his physician's blessing, he discontinued taking all of his heartburn medications, and his heartburn did not return.

• *Respiratory and allergy relief.* Other people state that their respiratory problems, including asthma and allergies, improved. Terry reported that his asthma and bronchitis symptoms improved to the point where he needed much less medication to control them.

• *Improved arthritis.* Whether it is from the decreased sugar intake or the fact that a lower weight reduces the stress on the joints, many arthritis sufferers have reported a decrease in their arthritis symptoms. Evette says that her flare-ups have been much less frequent since she adopted a low carbohydrate lifestyle.

• *Improved premenstrual syndrome (PMS).* Many women report an improvement in a number of the uncomfortable symptoms that plagued them before the start of their menstruation. Suzanne says that after her cycles became regular again (she experienced some irregularities when first beginning her diet), her tremendous PMS cravings were gone. From her perspective, that was just one of the "miracles" of reduced carbohydrate diets.

• *Improved polycystic ovarian syndrome (PCOS).* Several women who suffered from PCOS for years were quite surprised when their symptoms either greatly improved or disappeared altogether after they switched to a low carbohydrate lifestyle. Ciara reports that her symptoms "dramatically disappeared." She finds her symptoms are best controlled when she keeps her intake of carbohydrate at a fairly low level of about 20 grams per day. In fact, many physicians are recommending low carbohydrate diets to women with

PCOS who are trying to conceive. (For the web address of a PCOS support group for women who are trying to conceive, see Chapter 6.)

- *Improved fibromyalgia.* Many people who suffered for years with fibromyalgia report that their symptoms improved significantly after they began a reduced carbohydrate diet. Lucinda says her husband enjoyed dramatic improvements in his debilitating fibromyalgia after only two months on the diet.

- *Reduced yeast infections.* Many women who struggled with recurring yeast infections over the years find that their yeast infections either occur less frequently or have disappeared altogether.

- *Improved dental health.* Dentists have long warned of the detrimental effects of sugar on our teeth, and low carbohydrate dieters have confirmed the wisdom of their warnings. Many people report an improvement in the health of their gums since eliminating sugar from their diet. Brandi says she was plagued with chronic bleeding of her gums until she became a low carbohydrate dieter, at which point her gums healed.

- *Control of epileptic seizures.* In the 1920s, before the development of epileptic drugs such as Dilantin, ketogenic diets were routinely used to control seizures in epileptic patients. Since 1998, ketogenic diets have been making a comeback as a method to control seizures in people (mostly children) who have difficulty doing so with medications. In fact, Stanford University Medical School has a ketogenic diet program at Lucille Packard Children's Hospital, and Johns Hopkins University has a ketogenic diet program at its Epilepsy Center. (For links to web sites for these programs, see Chapter 6.)

- *A "new" wardrobe.* Nearly all of us have a section of

our closets reserved for the smaller clothes we hope to wear again. As she was packing for a trip, Callie decided to try on some of the clothes she had not worn for years. She found that she suddenly had a whole "new" wardrobe, and she was able to wear about a dozen smaller-sized shirts and pants again.

- *Fewer bees at picnics.* Now that you have eliminated sugar from your diet, bugs are much less likely to find your picnic lunch attractive!
- *Happier, fitter pets.* Many people report that their chubby, lazy family dog is now also getting regular workouts and has slimmed down and gained energy, too. Lena regularly posts her dog Nutball's weight loss progress along with hers. So far, Nutball has reduced his weight from 10.5 pounds to 8.5 pounds, a reduction of 19 percent of his body weight.
- *Happier, fitter kids.* The same benefits our pets are enjoying are being enjoyed by our kids, too!

Keep your own motivation log to remind you of all the benefits you have experienced since you began your reduced carbohydrate diet. Read it when you are frustrated with your weight loss to remind yourself that there are many reasons to stick with the reduced carbohydrate lifestyle. You might also want to keep pictures of yourself to document your progress.

Join an Internet Support Group

Join an Internet support group if you can. One of the key differences between the low carbohydrate diet revolution of the 1970s and the present revolution is that we now have easy access to the Internet. In the 1980s, when low fat dieting became the standard medical advice, few of us had access to dieting information other than through the popular media. Unfortunately, for 20 years, reduced carbohydrate dieting was not presented as a valid option in the media. The Internet changed everything in that it provided a fertile field in which the idea of reduced carbohydrate dieting could sprout and grow. The Internet has made it possible for reduced carbohydrate dieters to support one another and share their experiences. Their success stories have an unfettered and free outlet, and their testimonials are persuasive. There are now "virtual communities" made up of reduced carbohydrate web sites and message boards.

This wealth of readily available, unbiased information is one of the catalysts for the phenomenal growth of reduced carbohydrate diets. If you do not currently participate in one of these Internet groups, try to get on-line now. If you do not own a computer, check your local public library, which may have computers complete with Internet access.

The support and unbiased information you can receive from your reduced carbohydrate dieting peers will inspire you tremendously. These wonderful groups are a constant source of inspiration, motivation, and information. They are well worth the time and effort. For a list of Internet support groups, see Chapter 6.

Adjust Your Attitude

The final piece of advice from seasoned reduced carbohydrate dieters is to remember to be patient and to remind yourself that periods of slow weight loss are to be expected. You basically have two choices: You can continue your diet and be successful in the long run, or you can go back to your previous way of eating and risk regaining the weight you have lost thus far. For most of us, being stuck is a much better alternative than getting bigger.

Celebrate the weight you have already lost. Whether it is 5 pounds or 50 pounds, you should shift your focus from the weight that has yet to come off to the weight that has already departed.

Recognize that none of us achieve our weight loss goals without at least some trial and error. All of us stall, face temptation, lose some battles, and wonder if we are ever going to be able to look another egg in the eye. But we also whoosh, beat down temptations, and win victories. Many of us find that, overall, the road is much smoother than we ever thought possible and, after a while, eating low carbohydrate foods stops being a diet—it becomes a way of life. And that is when we know we will succeed.

5
Advice From the Experts

Now that we have covered the advice from the seasoned reduced carbohydrate dieters who have "been there and done that," let's take a look at the advice given by those who started it all—the reduced carbohydrate diet experts. As I am sure you recall from Chapter 1, each of these experts has his or her own perspective on the best ways to lose weight on reduced carbohydrate diets. When it comes to slow weight loss, stalls, and plateaus, it is much the same story, as they all have their individual theories on why they occur and how best to reverse them. While some of the experts agree some of the time, they each have their own unique approach.

This chapter presents brief summaries of the experts' opinions as they are presented in their books and on their web sites. These summaries are presented in alphabetical order according to the authors' last names. For an at-a-glance comparison of the experts' opinions, see Table 5.1 on pages 307–311.

Advice From Dr. Atkins (*Dr. Atkins' New Diet Revolution*)

In *Dr. Atkins' New Diet Revolution,* Dr. Atkins refers to people who have a difficult time losing weight, even on his plan, as being metabolically resistant. He addresses metabolic resistance in some detail in this book (he devotes a chapter to extreme metabolic resistance) and on his web site. For all of us, whether we are metabolically resistant or not, Dr. Atkins offers the following advice for avoiding pitfalls that can slow weight loss:

- *Too much carbohydrate.* Dr. Atkins states on his web site that he believes too much carbohydrate is the most common cause of slow weight loss. He advises us to be diligently attentive to the exact quantities of carbohydrates we eat. He cautions that overlooked and hidden carbohydrates are the most common reasons we underestimate our true carbohydrate intake. To ensure an accurate carbohydrate count, he recommends we document all the food we eat in a journal for at least several days. If our food journal does not reveal sources of hidden or overlooked carbohydrate that we can easily omit from our diet, he recommends we return to the Induction phase of the diet and eat 20 grams of carbohydrate or less per day for a week. He then instructs us to establish a new CCLL that allows our weight loss to continue.
- *Overeating.* While Dr. Atkins believes it is not necessary to count calories on his diet, he cautions that it is important to eat only until satisfied, not until stuffed. He also suggests eating at a slower pace to increase our satisfaction with eating. Eating more slowly also allows the "full" signal (generated by our stomachs) to

register in our brains before we overdo it and eat too much.

- *Undereating.* On the other end of the spectrum, he also warns that undereating will cause our bodies to resist losing weight. He advises us to eat when we are hungry and not to allow ourselves to get to the point where we feel as though we are starving.

- *Too little fat.* Dr. Atkins cautions against trying to combine his diet with low fat diets. In his judgment, restricting fat inhibits weight loss by reducing our satiety and leaving us more vulnerable to hunger and cravings. He also believes that when we eat fat without the presence of carbohydrate, the rate at which our bodies burn fat increases.

- *Nutritional deficiencies.* Dr. Atkins believes that nutritional deficiencies resulting from previous low calorie, low fat diets inhibit weight loss. He devotes an entire chapter of *Dr. Atkins' New Diet Revolution* to the subject. He firmly recommends a comprehensive multivitamin and a supplement of essential fatty acids as the *minimum* requirements for nutrient supplementation. He has developed his own line of nutritional supplements, known as Vita-Nutrients, which are specifically designed for low carbohydrate dieters.

- *Medications.* Dr. Atkins states that many medications slow weight loss, and in his experience, prescription medications pose the greatest challenges. However, he cautions us not to discontinue taking any prescription medications without the guidance of our personal physicians.

- *Yeast overgrowth.* Dr. Atkins is a strong advocate of the yeast overgrowth theory and believes that yeast overgrowth slows weight loss. In fact, he devotes an entire chapter of *Dr. Atkins' New Diet Revolution* to the subject. To combat yeast overgrowth, he recommends a version of his diet that omits yeast-containing foods, such as cheese, vinegar, wine, and mushrooms, for at least two weeks. He also recommends several nutritional supplements and medications to control yeast overgrowth.

- *Lack of exercise.* Dr. Atkins recommends that we engage in some type of exercise at least three times per week, or as directed by our physicians.

- *Lack of water.* Dr. Atkins recommends drinking at least eight glasses of water per day. He agrees with the purists who say that we should count only water (not water-based drinks) in our daily totals. He cautions that thirst is an indication we are not taking in enough water.

- *Underactive thyroid.* Dr. Atkins recommends that people whose body temperatures are consistently below normal get medical checkups. To determine if your body temperature is below normal, he recommends taking four temperature readings per day (before meals and at bedtime). If your average body temperature reading is below 97.8°F for three days or more, consult your physician about the possibility of an underactive thyroid.

- *Artificial sweeteners.* Dr. Atkins believes that most of us can use low to moderate amounts of artificial sweetener with little disruption in our rate of weight loss. However, he warns that overusing artificial sweeteners will slow weight loss, especially in people who are sensitive to them. He strongly discourages using aspartame and recommends using stevia or sucralose instead. He describes artificial sweeteners as "necessary evils" because they are much better alternatives than eating sugar when sugar cravings strike.

- *Caffeine.* Dr. Atkins believes that caffeine inhibits weight loss by causing our bodies to increase insulin production. He recommends consuming caffeine sparingly.
- *Alcohol.* Dr. Atkins believes that we should avoid drinking alcohol while on his diet. He believes alcohol slows weight loss because our bodies burn the alcohol as fuel rather than burning body fat stores. He states that if we choose to drink alcohol, we should limit our choices to low carbohydrate wines.
- *Hormone replacement therapy.* Dr. Atkins agrees that hormone replacement therapy, especially estrogen replacement, can slow weight loss. He recommends that women who are on hormone replacement therapy work with their physicians to evaluate natural alternatives.
- *Food intolerances.* Dr. Atkins devotes an entire chapter to the topic of how food intolerances can limit the effectiveness of his diet. He recommends rotating foods in and out of our diets to isolate their effects. Foods found to have negative effects should be eliminated.
- *The reversal diet.* Dr. Atkins recommends a technique he calls the reversal diet for breaking a plateau or controlling urges to abandon the diet. The technique is to go on another diet for a short period and then return to the Atkins diet. By doing so, some of us are able to regenerate the rapid weight loss we experienced early in the diet. However, there are a couple of limitations. First, going off the low carbohydrate diet is not an excuse to binge; Dr. Atkins instructs us to select a diet that restricts calories. Second, while it is acceptable to return to eating carbohydrate during this short break, we should continue to avoid simple sugars. Most of

our carbohydrate intake should continue to be in the form of complex carbohydrate.

- *Fat fast.* For those of us who suffer from extreme metabolic resistance, Dr. Atkins recommends a "fat fast," a technique in which food intake is restricted to macadamia nuts and cream cheese for a few days at a time. He cautions that only the unfortunate among us who have extreme metabolic resistance should use the fat fast. It should not be used simply to speed weight loss. The chapter of *Dr. Atkins' New Diet Revolution* that describes extreme metabolic resistance includes a full description of the fat fast technique.

Advice From Mr. Audette *(NeanderThin)*

Mr. Audette does not expressly discuss slow weight loss, stalls, or plateaus in his book *NeanderThin*. However, he does mention the following factors as they relate to the success of his diet:

- *Too much carbohydrate.* Mr. Audette cautions those of us who are using the NeanderThin diet for weight loss to limit the amount of fruit and other sources of carbohydrate, such as honey, that we eat. He says too much carbohydrate is the main reason for slow weight loss on his plan. He believes that people who wish to lose weight should get the majority of their calories from meats, nuts, seeds, and oils.
- *Forbidden foods.* Mr. Audette instructs us to completely abstain from eating the foods on his "forbidden foods" list, as he believes that eating them only causes us to crave more of them, particularly the carbohydrate in them.

- *Triggers.* Although he does not use this term to describe them, Mr. Audette warns us that alcohol and artificial sweeteners cause intense carbohydrate cravings.
- *Too little fat.* Mr. Audette cautions against restricting the amount of fat in our diets. He states that insufficient fat in our diet increases our hunger, lowers our metabolisms, and slows our overall weight loss.
- *Artificial sweeteners.* Mr. Audette believes that all sources of sweetness, including artificial sweeteners, slow our metabolic rates and our weight loss.
- *Alcohol.* Mr. Audette warns that alcohol causes us to intensely crave carbohydrate.
- *Water.* Mr. Audette believes that we should drink purified water, not tap water or any other fluids. He recommends drinking at least eight glasses of water a day, but prefers 2 to 4 liters (or more) a day.
- *Exercise.* Mr. Audette recommends engaging in regular, moderate activity, since it was important for the hunter-gatherer to walk to gather food. He does not think it necessary for us to engage in vigorous exercise to improve our health. He includes a five-week exercise program in his book.

Advice From the Eades *(Protein Power)*

Drs. Michael and Mary Dan Eades devote just a small amount of space in their book and on their web site to slow weight loss, stalls, and plateaus. They mention the following stumbling blocks:

- *Too much carbohydrate.* The Eades say the most common cause of slow weight loss and plateaus is too much carbohydrate in our diets. They instruct us to closely count our carbohydrate intake for a few days to uncover hidden carbohydrate and determine an accurate carbohydrate total. If we find we are losing very slowly or are stuck in a plateau while we are eating at (or below) the recommended 30 or 55 grams per day (depending on the diet phase), they recommend we cut our carbohydrate intake down to 10 to 20 grams per day for a few days.

- *Too many calories*. The Eades say that too much food is the second most common reason for slow weight loss and plateaus. They advise us to reduce the portion sizes of the foods we eat. In particular, they caution us not to overconsume cheese, nuts, or butter because these foods have high calorie counts. They instruct us to maintain our protein and carbohydrate counts at the levels recommended in their book. To reduce our calorie intake, the Eades recommend we cut our fat intake.

- *Lack of water*. The Eades recommend we drink at least 64 ounces of water per day, preferably immediately before meals. They define water as any water-based drink that does not contain carbohydrate or calories.

- *Too little protein*. The Eades caution that when our protein intake is below the minimum amount they recommend in their book, we lose lean body mass. They believe that losing lean body mass leads to a slowing of the metabolism, which in turn results in slowed weight loss.

- *Artificial sweeteners*. The Eades advise us that we should limit all artificial sweeteners to at least moderate levels and avoid aspartame altogether. They support the theory that artificial sweeteners can trigger

insulin releases and thereby cause carbohydrate cravings and hunger.

- *Too much protein.* While the Eades discount the theory that excess protein is readily converted to glucose
  and thereby produces weight loss stalls or weight gain,
  they do caution against exceeding the minimum protein requirements by a wide margin.
- *Vitamin deficiencies.* The Eades believe that nutritional deficiencies lead to hormonal imbalances and
  insulin resistance, which stall weight loss. They devote
  an entire chapter of *Protein Power* to the topic of nutritional supplements.
- *Caffeine.* The Eades do not believe caffeine is a problem for most of us, although they concede that some
  of us may be sensitive to it and may need to avoid it to
  be successful at weight loss.
- *Alcohol.* The Eades allow moderate alcohol intake on
  their plan, as long as we include the carbohydrate
  count in our daily totals. In fact, they believe that
  moderate wine intake is actually beneficial because it
  increases our bodies' sensitivity to insulin, thereby reducing insulin resistance. On the other hand, they believe that we should limit drinking distilled spirits
  because they can raise insulin levels and worsen
  insulin-related disorders. We should also avoid hard
  liquors, since they contribute empty calories to our
  diets.
- *Lack of exercise.* The Eades strongly believe that we
  benefit when we add exercise to our weight loss programs. They devote an entire chapter of *Protein Power*
  to the subject. They recommend strength training, as it
  builds lean body mass that, in turn, raises metabolism.
- *Underactive thyroid.* The Eades recommend that we
  seek thyroid evaluations from our physicians if we are

overweight, have elevated cholesterol levels, or are listless and without energy.

- *Estrogen replacement therapy*. The Eades advise women to take natural rather than synthetic estrogen. They believe that synthetic estrogen leaves women more prone to slow weight loss or weight gain. They also recommend that women work with their physicians to determine the lowest effective dose.

- *Smoking*. The authors state on their web site that they believe smoking promotes the development of insulin resistance and, therefore, we should avoid it.

Advice From the Hellers *(The Carbohydrate Addict's Diet)*

The Hellers briefly mention the topic of slow weight loss and plateaus in their book and on their web site. They claim plateaus are less frequent and of shorter duration on their diet than on the other reduced carbohydrate plans. They credit this relative lack of plateaus to the unique feature of the Reward Meal. They believe the Reward Meal prevents our bodies from going into starvation mode and slowing our metabolisms. They instruct us to weigh each day, but to track only our weekly averages as a measure of our progress. They discuss the following stumbling blocks in their book and on their web site:

- *Carbo drifting*. The Hellers state that "carbo drifting" is the most common reason for limited success on their plan. They use the term "carbo drifting" to describe what happens when we upset the balance of our Reward Meals by increasing the carbohydrate portion. In effect, eating too much carbohydrate in relation to the amount of protein and fat causes disruption of the balance of the Reward Meal.

- *Time limit.* The Hellers repeatedly caution that taking more than 60 minutes to eat the Reward Meal inhibits our weight loss.

- *Too much carbohydrate.* The Hellers caution us to analyze all the foods we eat in our Complementary Meals. They believe that even a small amount of carbohydrate-rich food or the consumption of hidden carbohydrate during the Complementary Meals slows our weight loss. They also caution us not to use protein powders during our Complementary Meals because these products contain several ingredients (most notably, artificial sweeteners) that stall weight loss.

- *Addiction triggers.* The Hellers advise us to also analyze all the foods we eat in our Complementary Meals to identify any potential triggers of unwanted insulin releases or addictive behaviors.

- *Too much food.* The Hellers suggest we reduce the amount of food we eat during our Complementary Meals as a way to break plateaus. They also suggest we skip Complementary Meals occasionally to reduce our overall food intake. However, they caution that we should never skip Reward Meals.

- *Artificial sweeteners.* The Hellers strongly believe that food and other substances that have a sweet taste, such as artificial sweeteners, are "carbohydrate act-alikes" that trick our bodies into releasing insulin as though we had eaten sugar. They strongly recommend that we omit all artificial sweeteners from the diet.

- *Monosodium glutamate (MSG).* The Hellers believe that MSG triggers insulin releases. They recommend identifying and avoiding all sources of MSG.

- *Caffeine.* Although the Hellers mention caffeine only

briefly in their book, they imply that it triggers carbo-hydrate cravings.

- *Water.* The Hellers recommend six to eight glasses of water per day.
- *Alcohol.* The Hellers recommend drinking alcohol only during Reward Meals.
- *Exercise.* While the Hellers say that exercise is not necessary on their diet, they do say that a moderate level of activity will enhance its effectiveness.

Advice From Dr. Pescatore *(Thin for Good)*

In *Thin for Good,* Dr. Pescatore gives the following advice related to factors he believes are the primary reasons people have difficulty losing weight on his plan:

- *Too much food.* Dr. Pescatore states that consuming too much food is the most common reason weight loss slows on his diet. He advises us to carefully watch the amount of food we eat, particularly of the foods he restricts.
- *Not enough food.* The second factor Dr. Pescatore mentions is overrestriction of the amount of food we eat. He cautions that undereating will lead to sluggish metabolism and slow weight loss.
- *Lack of water.* Dr. Pescatore states several times in his book that sufficient water intake is a vital factor in losing weight. His water rule is to drink "the amount of water in ounces that your body weighs in kilograms." (A pound equals 2.2 kilograms.) For example, a person who weighs 200 pounds should divide 200 by 2.2 and drink that amount of water in ounces per day (91 ounces in this example). He also believes that we

should consume water rather than other beverages, and he instructs us to exclude water-based drinks from our daily totals.

- *Lack of exercise.* Dr. Pescatore recommends regular, moderate exercise and devotes a chapter of the book to the subject.

- *Artificial sweeteners.* Dr. Pescatore warns that we should use artificial sweeteners, especially aspartame, sparingly. He agrees with the theory that the sweet taste of artificial sweeteners causes insulin releases and thereby stalls weight loss.

- *Yeast overgrowth.* Dr. Pescatore agrees that yeast overgrowth is a significant problem for many of us and believes it is one of the leading reasons for slow weight loss. He recommends consuming a modified diet minus yeast-containing foods and taking yeast-fighting supplements for at least three months.

- *Underactive thyroid.* Dr. Pescatore lists a sluggish thyroid as a common reason for slow weight loss. He instructs us to take our temperature with glass thermometers four times a day for at least four days. If our average body temperature is below 98°F, we should consult our physicians.

- *Food allergies.* Dr. Pescatore states that sensitivity to some foods can slow weight loss. He believes we become sensitive to a food when we have problems digesting or metabolizing it. He says we should keep food journals to determine if food allergies are a problem for us.

- *Hormone imbalances.* Although hormone imbalances can cause slow weight loss in either gender, Dr. Pescatore states they are more common in women. He recommends that women consult their physicians for full evaluations.

- *Hormone replacement therapy.* Dr. Pescatore mentions several times in his book that hormone replacement therapy can cause difficulties for women wishing to lose weight. However, he cautions women not to discontinue taking the drugs without guidance from their physicians.

- *Prescription drugs.* Dr. Pescatore agrees with the other reduced carbohydrate diet book authors who say that prescription drugs are a major cause of slow weight loss. However, he cautions us not to discontinue taking any prescription drugs without first consulting our physicians.

- *Nutritional deficiencies.* Dr. Pescatore is a strong believer that nutritional supplementation plays a vital role in losing weight. In fact, he devotes an entire chapter of his book to the topic.

- *Caffeine.* Dr. Pescatore agrees that caffeine causes an overproduction of insulin and should not be included in our diets.

- *Sodas.* Dr. Pescatore cautions us not to drink sodas, especially those containing aspartame.

- *Alcohol.* Dr. Pescatore recommends that we severely limit our consumption of alcohol while losing weight. He states that alcohol is metabolized by our bodies as a simple sugar and, therefore, should be avoided.

- *Gender differences.* Dr. Pescatore agrees that for many reasons, women lose weight more slowly than men. He offers a significant amount of advice in his book to women who are experiencing slow weight loss.

Advice From Dr. Schwarzbein *(The Schwarzbein Principle)*

Dr. Schwarzbein mentions slow weight loss only briefly in her book because she strongly recommends losing weight slowly; she believes there is no way to lose weight quickly and still remain healthy. However, she does discuss a few factors that she believes limit the success of her diet:

- *Caffeine.* Dr. Schwarzbein recommends removing caffeine from our diets. She supports the theory that caffeine triggers increased insulin levels.
- *Too few calories.* While she does not advocate the calorie theory for weight loss, Dr. Schwarzbein does state that taking in too little food will cause slowed metabolism and slowed weight loss.
- *Water.* Dr. Schwarzbein recommends drinking eight to ten glasses of water each day.
- *Exercise.* Dr. Schwarzbein states in her book that regular, moderate exercise is a critical piece of her plan and that exercise improves insulin resistance.
- *Artificial sweeteners.* Dr. Schwarzbein believes that artificial sweeteners, especially aspartame and saccharin, raise our insulin levels and should be excluded from our diets.
- *Alcohol.* Dr. Schwarzbein believes we should not drink alcohol because it raises our insulin levels.
- *Stimulants.* Dr. Schwarzbein strongly advises against using stimulants, including over-the-counter stimulants such as ephedrine, prescription stimulants, and illegal stimulants. She believes they deplete our critical serotonin levels and aggravate chemical imbalances.
- *Sodium.* Dr. Schwarzbein says we should not add salt

to our food because natural food sources provide sufficient amounts of it.

- *Vitamin deficiencies.* Dr. Schwarzbein believes the best sources of vitamins are natural, whole foods. Nonetheless, she discusses several nutritional supplements she believes are critical for optimal body function.
- *Hormone imbalances.* Dr. Schwarzbein advises us to get medical checkups to check for hormonal imbalances if we are not able to lose weight on her plan. She advises us to find physicians who prescribe real hormones rather than synthetic replacements.
- *Smoking.* Dr. Schwarzbein believes smoking contributes to insulin resistance, causes diabetes, and initiates insulin releases.

Advice From Dr. Sears *(The Zone)*

Dr. Sears briefly mentions the following issues related to slow weight loss and plateaus in his book and on his web sites:

- *Unfavorable carbohydrate.* Dr. Sears advises those of us who experience limited success on his plan to closely review our carbohydrate sources to ensure we are eating "favorable" carbohydrate such as low carbohydrate vegetables. He recommends low carbohydrate vegetables rather than fruits because they are less "carbohydrate dense."
- *Too much carbohydrate.* To speed weight loss, Dr. Sears recommends reducing the number of carbohydrate blocks we eat at each meal while increasing the number of fat blocks we eat. He states that this approach keeps our intake of calories at an adequate

level while decreasing the amount of insulin we release in response to the meal.

- *Too much protein.* Dr. Sears believes that eating protein stimulates the release of insulin, although to a much lesser degree than does eating carbohydrate. He believes that when we eat too much protein, we increase our insulin levels to the point that our weight loss stalls.

- *Not enough food.* Dr. Sears instructs us to make sure we take in enough carbohydrate, protein, and fat blocks per day.

- *Meal frequency and size.* Dr. Sears recommends dividing our food intake into small, frequent meals throughout the day.

- *Exercise.* Dr. Sears recommends increasing the amount of time we spend doing aerobic exercise.

- *Water.* Dr. Sears recommends that water be our primary beverage. He instructs us to drink at least eight glasses each day. He recommends drinking eight ounces with every meal. He recommends that we avoid beverages with calories, caffeine, or artificial sweeteners.

- *Artificial sweeteners.* Dr. Sears advocates that we eliminate artificial sweeteners from our diets. He believes artificial sweeteners cause rapid insulin releases and interfere with our success.

- *Caffeine.* Dr. Sears discourages caffeine use because he supports the theory that caffeine causes increased insulin levels.

- *Alcohol.* Dr. Sears believes that a moderate amount of alcohol enhances the production of good eicosanoids and is, therefore, beneficial. However, he warns that higher amounts lead to the production of bad eicosanoids. He recommends no more than one glass of wine per day.

- *Smoking.* Dr. Sears cites evidence that smoking leads to increased insulin levels and insulin resistance.
- *Ketosis.* Dr. Sears believes that ketosis leads to plateaus because the body reduces its metabolic rate in an effort to adjust to the "starvation" caused by the severe restriction of carbohydrate.

Advice From Mr. Steward et al.
(Sugar Busters!)

The topics of slow weight loss, stalls, and plateaus are not expressly mentioned in *Sugar Busters!* However, the authors offer several pieces of advice in the book and on their web site to enhance the success of their plan.

- *Too much carbohydrate.* Dr. Balart stated in an interview (posted on the Sugar Busters! web site) dated May 25, 1998, that people who have a difficult time losing weight on the plan should restrict their carbohydrate intake to foods that have a very low glycemic index.
- *Too much protein.* The authors caution us not to overeat protein. They state that excess protein is converted to glucose through glucogenesis and, therefore, raises our insulin levels and increases our body fat.
- *Alcohol.* The authors believe that our bodies use alcohol as fuel before using our stored body fat. Therefore, we will not lose weight after we drink alcohol. They state that we should drink red wine if we choose to drink. They also recommend drinking the alcohol on a full stomach. They believe the food digestion slows the alcohol absorption, thereby allowing us to release lesser amounts of insulin in response.

- *Caffeine.* The authors recommend limiting caffein-ated beverages to less than three cups per day. They believe caffeine stimulates our gastric acids and in-creases our appetites.
- *Water.* The authors recommend drinking six to eight glasses of water per day.
- *Exercise.* The authors recommend that we engage in moderate exercise. They caution us to avoid vigorous exercise because our bodies will produce the neces-sary energy by converting protein to glucose rather than using our body fat stores.
- *Meal frequency.* The authors believe eating at least three balanced meals a day will produce less insulin than eating one or two larger ones.

The authors devote a portion of *Sugar Busters!* to the unique challenges women face in losing weight. They dis-cuss the following reasons they believe women experience slower weight loss than men do:

- *Less exercise.* The authors believe that women exer-cise less than men. Further, they feel that when women do exercise, they tend to exercise less vigorously and aerobically than men do. They also believe men prac-tice more resistance training (weight lifting) and, therefore, build more muscle than women do.
- *More snacking.* The authors believe that women snack more than men, perhaps because they are usually in charge of food preparation.
- *Hormone medications.* Women are more likely to take hormone medications, such as birth control pills and progesterone replacement therapies. The authors state that progesterone increases appetite and promotes

weight gain. They state that, on the other hand, estrogen improves insulin sensitivity and may be beneficial.

- *Efficient fat storage.* The authors state that womens' bodies are more efficient at fat storage probably because of their reproductive role. They believe that female bodies are more adept at storing fat especially during and after pregnancies.

Table 5.1. Summary Table of the Experts' Advice

	Atkins	Audette	Eades	Hellers	Pescatore	Schwarzbein	Sears	Steward et al.
Too Much Carbohydrate	Main reason for slow loss; recommends food journal; watch for hidden carbohydrate; return to Induction	Main reason for slow loss; limit fruits and other sweets	Main reason for slow loss; recommends food journal; watch for hidden carbohydrate to 10–20 grams for a few days	Main reason for slow loss; keep to one-third of Reward Meal; restrict in Complementary Meals; recommends food journal	Main reason for limited success	Primary cause of obesity	Avoid "unfavorable" carbohydrate; recommends low glycemic index foods; reduce carbohydrate blocks and increase fat blocks at each meal and snack	Recommends restriction of carbohydrate to foods with a very low glycemic index
Overeating	Eat until satisfied, not stuffed; eat at slower pace	Does not address as a cause of slow loss	Second reason for slow loss; reduce fat; keep protein and carbohydrate at recommended levels	Do not eat beyond the 60-minute limit of Reward Meal; limit or skip Complementary Meals; do not limit or skip Reward Meals	Recommends portion control; provides serving size information in the list of allowed foods	Believes too much carbohydrate leads to overeating	Recommends calorie restriction: 500 calories or less per meal and 100 calories or less per snack	Recommends portion control; limit the amount of food to that which will fit on flat part of dinner plate
Too Much Protein	Does not address as a cause of slow loss	Does not address as a cause of slow loss	Do not exceed minimum protein requirement by a wide margin	Does not address as a cause of slow loss	Does not address as a cause of slow loss	Believes we have a mechanism that naturally limits our consumption of protein	Believes extra protein causes insulin releases and slows weight loss	Too much protein slows weight loss

Table 5.1. Summary Table of the Experts' Advice (Cont.)

	Atkins	Audette	Eades	Hellers	Pescatore	Schwarzbein	Sears	Steward et al.
Undereating	Do not wait until starving; eat when hungry	Does not address as a cause of slow loss	Ensure minimum intake of required protein	Does not address as a cause of slow loss	Ensure adequate intake to prevent slowed metabolism	Ensure adequate food intake; eat when hungry	Ensure adequate number of food blocks per day	Does not address as a cause of slow loss
Too Little Fat	Fat improves taste and satiety; without carbohydrate, fat increases rate of body fat breakdown	Lack of fat increases hunger, lowers metabolism, and slows weight loss	Does not address as a cause of slow loss	Does not address as a cause of slow loss	Does not address as a cause of slow loss	Does not address as a cause of slow loss, but advocates unrestricted intake of healthy fats	Does not agree that too little fat is a cause of slow loss	Does not agree that too little fat is a cause of slow loss
Addiction Triggers	Does not address as a cause of slow loss	Believes alcohol and artificial sweeteners create carbohydrate cravings	Does not address as a cause of slow loss	Recommends analyzing foods and situations to identify triggers	Does not address as a cause of slow loss	Does not address as a cause of slow loss, but believes sugar is addictive	Does not address as a cause of slow loss	Does not address as a cause of slow loss
Nutritional Deficiencies	Caused by improper previous diet; strong advocate of nutritional supplements	Does not address as a cause of slow loss	Contribute to insulin resistance and metabolic disturbances	Does not address as a cause of slow loss	Does not address as a Strong advocate of nutritional supplements	Strong emphasis on importance of adequate nutrients	Does not address as a cause of slow loss	Does not address as a cause of slow loss
Medications	Over-the-counter and prescription drugs cause slow	Does not address as a cause of slow loss	See "Hormone Imbalances and Hormone Replacement	Does not address as a cause of slow loss	Prescription drugs most troublesome; do not dis-	Does not address as a cause of slow	Does not address as a cause of slow	See "Hormone Imbalances and Hormone

Table 5.1. Summary Table of the Experts' Advice (Cont.)

	Atkins	Audette	Eades	Hellers	Pescatore	Schwarzbein	Sears	Steward et al.
	loss; do not discontinue without physician guidance		Therapy (HRT)"		continue without physician guidance	loss	loss	Replacement Therapy (HRT)"
Yeast Overgrowth	Recommends yeast-free diet, drugs and supplements	Does not address as a cause of slow loss	Does not address as a cause of slow loss	Does not address as a cause of slow loss	Recommends yeast-free diet and supplements	Does not address as a cause of slow loss	Does not address as a cause of slow loss	Does not address as a cause of slow loss
Exercise	Moderate exercise three times a week; devotes a chapter to the topic	Moderate; includes an exercise plan in book	Moderate; recommends strength training; devotes a chapter to the topic	Moderate; not required	Moderate; devotes a chapter to the topic	Moderate; devotes a chapter to the topic	Recommends; devotes a chapter to the topic; increase aerobic exercise	Moderate; caution vigorous exercise will cause glucogenesis
Water	Drink 8 glasses of water a day; no substitutes	Drink 8 glasses minimum of water a day; prefers 2–4 liters of purified water; no substitutes	Drink 64 ounces a day; includes water-based drinks without calories	Drink 6–8 glasses a day	Drink number of ounces that equals body weight in kilograms	Drink 8–10 glasses of water a day	Drink 8 glasses of water a day; no substitutes	Drink 6–8 glasses a day
Underactive Thyroid	Recommends a medical checkup if body temperature is below	Does not address as a cause of slow loss	Recommends thyroid evaluation	Does not address as a cause of slow loss	Recommends a medical checkup if body temperature is below	Does not address as a cause of slow loss	Does not address as a cause of slow loss	Does not address as a cause of slow loss

Table 5.1. Summary Table of the Experts' Advice (Cont.)

	Atkins	Audette	Eades	Hellers	Pescatore	Schwarzbein	Sears	Steward et al.
	97.8°F for several days				98.6°F for several days			
Artificial Sweeteners	Limit use of all artificial sweeteners; omit aspartame; prefers stevia or sucralose	Avoid use of all artificial sweeteners	Limit use of all artificial sweeteners; omit aspartame	Omit use of all artificial sweeteners	Use sparingly; omit aspartame; prefers stevia	Exclude from diet	Exclude from diet; causes insulin production	Does not address as a cause of slow loss
Caffeine	Omit from diet; causes insulin releases	Does not address as a cause of slow loss	No need to limit unless sensitive to it	Limit; can be trigger for cravings	Omit from diet; causes insulin releases	Omit caffeine (and all other stimulants) from diet; raises insulin levels and depletes serotonin	Omit from diet; causes insulin releases	Limit to three beverages per day; stimulates the appetite
Alcohol	Avoid; body will use as fuel rather than fat stores	Avoid; causes intense carbohydrate cravings	Moderate intake; wine beneficial for insulin sensitivity	Only at Reward Meals	Severely limit intake; body metabolizes as a simple sugar	Omit from diet; raises insulin levels	Wine beneficial; limit to 1 glass per day	Avoid; body will use as fuel rather than fat stores
Hormone Imbalances and Hormone Replacement Therapy (HRT)	Believes HRT slows weight loss; work with physician to find natural alternatives	Does not address as a cause of slow loss	Believes HRT slows weight loss; recommends natural sources of estrogen; reduce to minimum effective amount	Does not address as a cause of slow loss	Believes hormonal imbalances cause slow loss; work with physician to find alternatives	Believes hormonal imbalances cause slow loss; work with physician to find alternatives	Believes hormonal imbalances are major factors in obesity	Believes HRT slows weight loss

Table 5.1. Summary Table of the Experts' Advice (Cont.)

	Atkins	Audette	Eades	Hellers	Pescatore	Schwarzbein	Sears	Steward et al.
Smoking	Does not address as a cause of slow loss	Does not address as a cause of slow loss	Quit; smoking contributes to insulin resistance	Does not address as a cause of slow loss	Does not address as a cause of slow loss	Quit; smoking contributes to insulin resistance and diabetes	Quit; smoking contributes to insulin resistance	Does not address as a cause of slow loss
Food Intolerances	Rotate foods to identify food intolerances; omit offending foods	Does not address as a cause of slow loss	Does not address as a cause of slow loss	Does not address as a cause of slow loss	Keep food journal to identify food allergies; omit offending foods	Does not address as a cause of slow loss, but has a long list of foods to avoid	Does not address as a cause of slow loss	Does not address as a cause of slow loss
Other Factors	Reversal diet (go off diet and onto calorie-restricted diet for a few days) to rejuvenate weight loss Recommends fat fast only for those very metabolically resistant to losing weight	Eating forbidden foods slows loss		Monosodium glutamate slows loss	Remove soft drinks from diet, especially those that contain aspartame Believes women lose weight slower than men and therefore offers significant advice for women			Believes women lose weight slower than men because they snack more, exercise less, take HRT, and are more efficient at fat storage

6
Reduced Carbohydrate Diet Resources

In the early days of reduced carbohydrate dieting, we low carbohydrate dieters had very few resources available to us. With the exception of one or two excellent books, we had few places to turn for information, support, and products. All that has changed. We now have a wonderful array of books, audiocassettes, compact discs, web sites, retail and on-line stores, and newsletters. This chapter outlines some of the currently available resources; others are being added each day.

A word of caution: The inclusion of a resource here should not be interpreted as an endorsement of it. No claim is made here as to the quality, integrity, security, or performance of any site or product. As is true with all Internet sites, the web pages mentioned here should be approached with a bit of caution.

Resources From the Diet Experts

This section presents the resources provided by the diet experts. They are listed in alphabetical order by the experts' names. The books listed are those that are available in retail bookstores and on the experts' web sites. The

Amazon.com and Barnes & Noble (bn.com) web sites feature customer reviews of the books. Out-of-print books from these experts can also be accessed through several of these sites.

Dr. Robert C. Atkins

The Atkins Center for Complementary Medicine
150 East 55th Street
New York, NY 10022
(888) 285-4678

Books

> *Dr. Atkins' Diet Revolution* (New York: Bantam Books, 1973)
>
> *Dr. Atkins' Health Revolution: How Complementary Medicine Can Extend Your Life* (New York: Bantam Books, 1990)
>
> *Dr. Atkins' New Diet Revolution* (New York: Avon Books, 1992)
>
> *Dr. Atkins' New Diet Cookbook* (New York: M. Evans and Company, 1994)
>
> *Dr. Atkins' Quick and Easy New Diet Cookbook* (New York: Fireside, 1997)
>
> *Dr. Atkins' New Carbohydrate Gram Counter* (New York: M. Evans and Company, 1997)
>
> *Dr. Atkins' New Diet Revolution,* revised and updated (New York: Avon, 1998)
>
> *Dr. Atkins' Vita-Nutrient Solution: Nature's Answer to Drugs* (New York: Fireside, 1998)
>
> *Dr. Atkins' Age-Defying Diet Revolution* (New York: St. Martin's Press, 2000)

Audiocassettes and Videotapes

Dr. Atkins' New Diet Revolution, two audiocassettes (Harper Audio, 1998)

Atkins' Answers, two videotapes with workbook (Ventura, 1999)

Dr. Atkins' Age-Defying Diet Revolution, audiobook (Simon & Schuster, 2000)

Official Web Site

http://www.atkinscenter.com

This is the official web site for the Atkins Center for Complementary Medicine in New York City. This web site has the following features:

- A summary of low carbohydrate diet news and articles
- A listing of scheduled appearances by Dr. Atkins
- A summary of the Atkins diet
- Answers to frequently asked questions (with a searchable database)
- An electronic mailbox that allows visitors to ask questions
- Information about the Atkins Center including phone number and address
- Information about the medical treatments offered at the Atkins Center
- An on-line store for Atkins books, foods, supplements, and products
- A search tool to locate retailers who carry Atkins products

Newsletter

> Dr. Atkins' Health Revelations Newsletter

Magazine

> Atkins: A Passion for Healthy Living

Mr. Ray Audette

Books

> NeanderThin: Eat Like a Caveman to Achieve a Lean, Strong, Healthy Body (New York: St. Martin's Press, 1999)

Official Web Site

http://www.neanderthin.com

This is the official web site for NeanderThin. The web site has the following features:

- A summary of Paleolithic nutrition
- Answers to frequently asked questions
- How to schedule Mr. Audette for lectures
- The *NeanderThin* bibliography
- Articles about Paleolithic nutrition
- Links to other Paleolithic web sites
- Media clips
- Bookstore to buy *NeanderThin*
- Paleolithic resources

Dr. Richard K. Bernstein

Book

> The Diabetes Solution: The Complete Guide to Achieving Normal Blood Sugars (Boston: Little, Brown and Company, 1997)

Official Web Site

http://www.diabetes-normalsugars.com

This is the official web site for Dr. Bernstein. The web site has the following features:

- A summary of Dr. Bernstein's diet
- Summaries of other low carbohydrate and moderate carbohydrate diets
- Answers to frequently asked questions
- Low carbohydrate recipes
- Articles
- Links to other diabetic and low carbohydrate web sites
- Bookstore to buy Dr. Bernstein's book

Dr. Michael Eades and Dr. Mary Dan Eades

The Colorado Center for Metabolic Medicine
7490 Clubhouse Road #103
Boulder, CO 80301-3720
(303) 530-5555

Books

Protein Power: The High-Protein/Low Carbohydrate Way to Lose Weight, Feel Fit, and Boost Your Health—In Just Weeks! (New York: Bantam Books, 1997)

The Protein Power LifePlan Gram Counter (New York: Warner Books, 2000)

The Doctor's Complete Guide to Vitamins and Minerals (New York: Dell Publishing Company, 2000)

The Protein Power LifePlan: A New Comprehensive Blueprint for Optimal Health (New York: Warner Books, 2001)

Audiocassette

The Protein Power LifePlan: A New Comprehensive Blueprint for Optimal Health (Time Warner Audio Books, 2000)

Official Web Sites

The Eades maintain two web sites related to *Protein Power.*

http://www.eatprotein.com

This is the official web site for the Colorado Center for Metabolic Medicine in Boulder, Colorado. This web site has the following features:

- A summary of low carbohydrate diet articles and books. The *Protein Power* bibliography
- Answers to frequently asked questions
- An electronic mailbox that allows visitors to ask questions

- A summary of the Protein Power diet
- A discussion group message board
- Free on-line recipes
- Information about the Colorado Center
- An on-line store for Protein Power books, foods, supplements, and products

http://www.proteinpower.com

This is the official web site for Protein Power products. The web site has the following features:

- Biographies of Drs. Michael and Mary Dan Eades
- Answers to frequently asked questions
- An on line store for Protein Power books, foods, supplements, and products
- A "members only" club of Protein Power products
- Success stories

Newsletter

Nutritional Wisdom, an e-mail newsletter is available at http://www.eatprotein.com.

Dr. Rachael Heller and Dr. Richard Heller

The Carbohydrate Addict's Center
Mount Sinai School of Medicine
Box 1194
New York, NY 10029

Books

The Carbohydrate Addict's Diet: The Lifelong Solution to Yo-Yo Dieting (New York: Signet, 1993)

The Carbohydrate Addict's Program for Success: Taking Charge of Your Life and Your Weight, companion workbook (New York: Plume, 1993)

The Carbohydrate Addict's Healthy for Life (New York: Plume, 1996)

The Carbohydrate Addict's LifeSpan Program: A Personalized Plan for Becoming Slim, Fit and Healthy in your 40s, 50s, 60s and Beyond (New York: Plume, 1997)

Carbohydrate-Addicted Kids: Help Your Child or Teen Break Free of Junk Food and Sugar Cravings—For Life! (New York: HarperPerennial, 1997)

The Carbohydrate Addict's Healthy Heart Program: Break Your Carbo-Insulin Connection to Heart Disease (New York: Ballantine Books, 1999)

The Carbohydrate Addict's Carbohydrate Counter (New York: Signet, 2000)

The Carbohydrate Addict's Calorie Counter (New York: Signet, 2000)

The Carbohydrate Addict's Fat Counter (New York: Signet, 2000)

The Carbohydrate Addict's Gram Counter (New York: Signet, 2000)

The Carbohydrate Addict's Cookbook: 250 All-New Low-Carb Recipes That Will Cut the Cravings and Keep You Slim for Life (New York: John Wiley & Sons, 2001)

Official Web Site

http://www.carbohydrateaddicts.com

This is the official web site for the Carbohydrate Addict's Diet programs. This web site has the following features:

- A summary of the Carbohydrate Addict's Diet for adults and kids
- Answers to frequently asked questions
- A quiz to determine the degree of carbohydrate addiction
- Discussion group message board via e-mail
- Discussion group live chat room
- An on-line store for Carbohydrate Addict's Diet books
- Success stories

Dr. Fred Pescatore

Books

Thin for Good: The One Low-Carb Diet That Will Finally Work for You (New York: John Wiley & Sons, 2000)
Feed Your Kids Well: How to Help Your Child Lose Weight and Get Healthy (New York: John Wiley & Sons, 2000)

Dr. Diana Schwarzbein

Books

The Schwarzbein Principle: The Truth About Losing Weight, Being Healthy, and Feeling Younger (Deerfield Beach, FL: Health Communications, 1999)

The Schwarzbein Principle Cookbook (Deerfield Beach, FL: Health Communications, 1999)

The Schwarzbein Principle Vegetarian Cookbook (Deerfield Beach, FL: Health Communications, 1999)

Dr. Barry Sears

Eicotech
21 Tioga Way
Marblehead, MA 01915

Books

The Zone: A Dietary Road Map to Lose Weight Permanently, Reset Your Genetic Code, Prevent Disease, Achieve Maximum Physical Performance (New York: HarperCollins, 1995)

Mastering the Zone: The Next Step in Achieving Superhealth and Permanent Fat Loss (New York: HarperCollins, 1996)

Zone Perfect Meals in Minutes (New York: HarperCollins, 1997)

Zone Food Blocks: The Quick and Easy, Mix and Match Counter for Staying in the Zone (New York: Regan Books, 1998)

The Anti-Aging Zone (New York: HarperCollins, 1998)

Starch Madness (Nevada City, CA: Blue Dolphin Publishing, 1999)

A Week in the Zone (New York: Regan Books, 2000)

The Top 100 Zone Foods: Supercharge Your Health (New York: Regan Books, 2000)

The Age-Free Zone (New York: Regan Books, 2000)

Great Food in the Zone (New York: HarperCollins, 2001)

The Soy Zone: 101 Delicious and Easy-to-Prepare Recipes (New York: Regan Books, 2001)

Audiocassettes

The Zone: A Dietary Road Map to Lose Weight Permanently, Reset Your Genetic Code, Prevent Disease, Achieve Maximum Physical Performance (Harper Audio, 1995)

Mastering the Zone: The Next Step in Achieving Superhealth and Permanent Fat Loss (Harper Audio, 1997)

The Zone Audio Collection (Harper Audio, 1997)

The Anti-Aging Zone (HarperCollins, 1999)

Official Web Sites

Dr. Sears maintains two web sites related to *The Zone*.

http://www.drsears.com

This is one of the official web sites for Dr. Barry Sears and the Zone diet. This web site has the following features:

- A summary of the Zone diet
- A summary of Zone diet news, articles, and research
- *The Zone* and *The Anti-Aging Zone* bibliographies
- A listing of scheduled appearances by Dr. Sears
- Answers to frequently asked questions
- An electronic mailbox that allows visitors to ask questions
- A searchable database
- A discussion group message board
- Free on-line recipes

- Success stories and testimonials
- A body fat calculator
- Zone food block guide
- Glycemic index information
- Restaurant information, including for fast-food restaurants
- Exercise information
- Carbohydrate information
- On-line store for Zone books, foods, supplements, and products

http://www.perfectzone.com

This is the second official web site for Dr. Barry Sears and the Zone diet. It is very similar to the first site and has the following features:

- A summary of the Zone diet
- A summary of Zone diet news, articles, and research
- A discussion group message board
- Free on-line recipes
- Success stories and testimonials
- A body fat calculator
- Zone links
- On-line store for Zone books, foods, supplements, and products
- Retail locator for Zone products
- Course for certifications to become a Zone-certified instructor

Mr. H. Leighton Steward, Dr. Morrison C. Bethea, Dr. Sam S. Andrews, and Dr. Luis A. Balart

Books

Sugar Busters! Cut Sugar to Trim Fat (New York: Ballantine Books, 1998)

Sugar Busters! Shopper's Guide (New York: Random House, 1999)

Sugar Busters! Quick and Easy Cookbook (New York: Ballantine Books, 1999)

Sugar Busters! for Kids (New York: Ballantine Books, 2001)

Audiocassette

Sugar Busters! Cut Sugar to Trim Fat (HarperCollins, 1998)

Official Web Site

http://www.sugarbusters.com

This is the official web site for the Sugar Busters! diet plan. This web site has the following features:

- A summary of reduced carbohydrate diet news and articles
- A summary of the Sugar Busters! diet plan
- Author biographies
- Several interviews with the authors
- Answers to frequently asked questions
- Discussion group message board
- Discussion group live chat room
- A searchable database

- An on-line store for Sugar Busters! books and foods
- A list of customer reviews
- A customer survey

Internet Support Groups

This section presents web sites that host reduced carbohydrate discussion groups. In addition to message boards, many of these web sites have other helpful features, such as recipes, on-line stores, and related information of all kind. These web sites are presented in alphabetical order by the site name.

Although many of these web sites use the names of the diet experts, they are not official web sites unless noted. Many of these web sites are owned and controlled by individuals who successfully lost weight with reduced carbohydrate dieting and wish to support the movement. For the most part, these individuals are not experts. While these web sites are wonderful sources of unbiased support and information, it is important to remember they are open, unmonitored forums. With the exception of profanity and abusive language, participants can post anything they wish.

As is true when participating in any Internet discussion group, protection of privacy may be a concern. It is a common practice for participants to use secondary electronic mailboxes and fictitious names when participating in a group. You may wish to do the same, at least until you become accustomed to the group.

Mixed Discussion Groups

The following general discussion groups are mixed groups in that they are not oriented to any one reduced carbohydrate diet plan.

Site name: alt.support.diet.low-carb
Site address: http://www.grossweb.com/asdlc/
Site features: A very active message board (America On-Line keyword "Newsgroups")

Site name: Carb Health
Site address: http://www.e-clipse.com
Site features:

- Message board
- Chat room
- Links to other low carbohydrate web sites
- Recipes and menu planners
- Book and low carbohydrate product store
- Product reviews
- Newsletter (e-mail)
- Success stories and testimonials

Site name: Florida Lowcarb Corner
Site address: http://www.se.mediaone.net/~zibbler/LC_home.htm
Site features:

- Message board
- Links to other low carbohydrate sites
- Recipes
- Book and low carbohydrate product store
- Diet tips

Site name: ivillage.com
Site address: http://www.ivillage.com/diet/boards/
Site features:

- Several message boards on a variety of topics including low carbohydrate dieting
- Recipes
- Fitness information
- Fitness product reviews
- A large variety of diet and fitness information

Site name: LivingSlim.com
Site address: http://www.livingslim.com
Site features:

- Message board
- Recipes
- Weight tracker
- Diet tips
- Medical information
- Testimonials

Site name: The Low Carb Cafe
Site address: http://www.lowcarbcafe.com
Site features:

- Message board
- Chat room
- Summaries of the major reduced carbohydrate diets
- Directory of and links to other low carbohydrate web sites
- Recipes
- Book and low carbohydrate product store
- Carbohydrate counter

Site name: Low Carb Pavilion
Site address: http://wilstar.com/lowcarb
Site features:

- Message board
- Brief explanation of low carbohydrate diets
- Links to several low carbohydrate web sites
- Low carbohydrate product store
- Summary of supportive low carbohydrate research
- Hidden carbohydrate information
- Nutrition chemistry information
- Food pyramid information
- Listing of low carbohydrate resources
- Health news

Site name: Low-Carb Diet Information Clearinghouse
Site address: http://www.lowcarb.ca
Site features:

- Message board
- Recipes
- News and research
- Diet tips
- Success stories and testimonials
- Book and low carbohydrate product store

Site name: Lowcarb Mailing Lists
Site address: http://members.aol.com/lowcarbs/index.htm
Site features:

- Links to several low carbohydrate mailing lists
- Instructions on how to subscribe and unsubscribe to
  the lists

Site name: LowCarbEating.com
Site address: http://lowcarbeating.com
Site features:

- Message board
- Chat room
- Overview of low carbohydrate dieting basics
- Recipes
- Shopping tips
- Product reviews
- Books and products store
- Newsletter

Site name: LoCarbLosers
Site address: http://groups.yahoo.com/group/locarblosers
Site features:
- Message board

Site name: Oprah.com (official web site of *Oprah*)
Site address: http://oprah.com
Site features:

- Several message boards on a variety of health-related topics including low carbohydrate dieting
- Recipes

Site name: Thinner.com
Site address: http://www.thinner.com
Site features:

- Message board
- Chat room
- Recipes
- Links to other low carbohydrate web sites

- Searchable message board archives
- Success stories
- Product store
- Free electronic mailbox

Site name: 3 Fat Chicks on a Diet!
Site address: http://www.3fatchicks.com
Site features:

- Message board
- Chat room
- Newsletter (e-mail)
- Book reviews
- Recipes
- Fast-food guide
- Links to other low carbohydrate sites
- Food reviews

Site name: Vegetarian Lowcarb
Site address: http://www.immuneweb.org/lowcarb
Site features:

- Message mailing list
- Recipes and menus
- Articles and resources
- Links to other low carbohydrate web sites
- Searchable message board archives
- Product store

Atkins Diet Support Groups

Site name: Atkins & Low Carb Friends.com
Site address: http://atkinsfriends.com

Site features:

- Message board
- Chat room
- Answers to frequently asked questions
- Recipes
- Carbohydrate counter
- Atkins news
- Calendar of events
- Product store
- Links to other low carbohydrate web sites
- Polls and surveys (with searchable archives)
- Success stories
- Glossary of terms
- Greeting cards
- Friends tracker
- Gaming area
- Humor

Site name: Atkins and Low Carb Support Forum
Site address: http://communities.msn.com/
AtkinsandLowCarbsupportforum
Site features:

- Message board
- Chat room
- Recipes
- Links to Atkins sites
- Photo album

Site name: Atkins Chat.com
Site address: http://www.atkinschat.com

Site features:

- Message board
- E-mail list
- Chat room
- Recipes
- Carbohydrate counts

Site name: The Atkins Diet Help.com
Site address: http://www.atkinsdiethelp.com
Site features:

- Message board
- Recipes
- Answers to frequently asked questions
- News
- Success stories
- Bookstore
- Supplement shop
- Common carbohydrate counter
- Searchable message board archives

Site name: Everything Atkins
Site address: http://www7.addr.com/~atkinsdiet
Site features:

- Message board
- Chat room
- Recipes
- Diet tips
- Bookstore
- Reference section

Site name: ivillage.com
Site address: http://www.ivillage.com/diet/boards/
Site features:

- Message board
- Recipes
- Fitness information
- Fitness product reviews
- A large variety of diet and fitness information

Carbohydrate Addict's Diet Support Groups

Site name: Carbohydrate Addict's Network (official web site
of the Carbohydrate Addict's Program)
Site address: http://www.carbohydrateaddicts.com
Site features:

- Message board
- Chat room
- Answers to frequently asked questions
- Recipes
- Carbohydrate Addict's Diet summary
- Information for adults and kids
- A quiz to determine the degree of carbohydrate addiction
- Carbohydrate Addict's Bookstore
- Success stories

Site name: ivillage.com
Site address: http://www.ivillage.com/diet/boards/
Site features:

- Message board
- Recipes

- Fitness information
- Fitness product reviews
- A large variety of diet and fitness information

Protein Power Diet Support Groups

Site name: ivillage.com
Site address: http://www.ivillage.com/diet/boards/
Site features:

- Message board
- Recipes
- Fitness information
- Fitness product reviews
- A large variety of diet and fitness information

Site name: Protein Power (official web site of Protein Power)
Site address: http://www.eatprotein.com
Site features:

- Message board
- Recipes
- Answers to frequently asked questions
- An electronic mailbox that allows visitors to ask questions of the Drs. Eades
- Protein Power diet summary
- Low carbohydrate article summaries
- The *Protein Power* bibliography
- Store for food, supplements, and Protein Power products

Sugar Busters! Diet Support Groups

Site name: Sugar Busters!.com (official site of Sugar Busters!)
Site address: http://www.sugarbusters.com
Site features:

- Message board
- Chat room
- Answers to frequently asked questions
- News and articles
- Sugar Busters! diet plan summary
- Author biographies
- Authors' interviews
- A searchable database
- Store for Sugar Busters! products
- Customer reviews
- Customer survey

The Zone Diet Support Groups

Site name: drsears.com (official site of the Zone diet)
Site address: http://www.drsears.com
Site features:

- Message board
- Answers to frequently asked questions
- Recipes
- Zone diet summary and comparisons to other diet programs
- Zone news, articles, and research
- A listing of scheduled appearances by Dr. Sears
- An electronic mailbox that allows visitors to ask questions

- A searchable database
- Success stories and testimonials
- A body fat calculator
- Zone food block guide
- Restaurant information, including fast-food restaurants
- Exercise information
- Carbohydrate information
- Store for Zone books, foods, supplements, and products

Site name: ivillage.com
Site address: http://www.ivillage.com/diet/boards/
Site features:

- Message board
- Recipes
- Fitness information
- Fitness product reviews
- A large variety of diet and fitness information

Site name: Zone Home
Site address: http://www.zonehome.com
Site features:

- Message board
- Answers to frequently asked questions
- Recipes
- Zone diet summary
- Store for Zone books, products, and services
- Site searches
- Library of recommended books
- Links to other health-related web sites
- Find a friend

Site name: Zone Perfect.com (official site of The Zone diet)
Site address: http://zoneperfect.com
Site features:

- Message board
- Answers to frequently asked questions
- Recipes
- Zone diet summary
- Zone news, articles, and research
- An electronic mailbox that allows visitors to ask questions
- Success stories and testimonials
- Restaurant information, including fast-food restaurants
- Exercise information
- Carbohydrate information
- Store for Zone books, foods, supplements, and products
- E-mail newsletter
- ZonePerfect Club

Cookbooks and Recipes

In the early days of reduced carbohydrate dieting, one of the most common criticisms was that it was boring. It had an undeserved reputation as a "meat-and-cheese diet." One of the really great developments in reduced carbohydrate dieting is the current proliferation of low carbohydrate cookbooks and Internet recipe sites. These new cookbooks and recipe sites have spawned a whole new genre of cooking that supports us in our quest to lose weight.

Cookbooks Available in Bookstores

The following cookbooks are listed in alphabetical order by author's name. The Amazon.com and Barnes and Noble (bn.com) web sites contain customer reviews that may be helpful in making a selection. Many libraries also carry the books.

Atkins, Robert C., and Veronica Atkins. *Dr. Atkins' Quick and Easy New Diet Cookbook*. New York: Fireside Books, 1997.

Bahan, Deanie Comeaux. *Sugarfree New Orleans: A Cookbook Based on the Glycemic Index*. New Orleans: AFM Publishing, 1997.

Chud, Deborah Friedman. *The Gourmet Prescription: High Flavor Recipes for Lower Carbohydrate Diets*. Coronado, CA: Bay Books, 1999.

Doyen, Barbara Hartsock. *Back to Protein: The Low Carb, No Carb Meat Cookbook*. New York: M. Evans and Company, 2000.

Haas, Alex. *Everyday Low Carb Cookery*, revised edition. Fall River, MA: Alex Haas, 1999.

Heller, Richard. *The Carbohydrate Addict's Cookbook: 250 All-New Low-Carb Recipes That Will Cut the Cravings and Keep You Slim for Life*. New York: John Wiley & Sons, 2001.

McCullough, Fran. *The Low-Carb Cookbook: The Complete Guide to the Healthy Low-Carbohydrate Lifestyle With Over 250 Delicious Recipes*. New York: Hyperion, 1997.

Randolph, Lauri Ann. *Lauri's Low-Carb Cookbook: Rapid Weight Loss with Satisfying Meals!*, second edition. New York: Avalon Enterprises, 1999.

Rayburn, Linda. *Living (and Loving) the Low-Carb Life!* Np: Darlin Publications, 1999.

Ross, Tami, and Patti Geil. *The Carbohydrate Counting Cookbook*. New York: John Wiley & Sons, 1998.

Schwarzbein, Diana. *The Schwarzbein Principle Cookbook*. Deerfield Beach, FL: Health Communications, 1999.

Schwarzbein, Diana. *The Schwarzbein Principle Vegetarian Cookbook*. Deerfield Beach, FL: Health Communications, 1999.

Schweinhart, Belinda, and Chaddie Letson. *Low Carb Recipes Fast & Easy*. Self-published, 1999.

Steward, H. Leighton; Morrison Bethea; Sam Andrews; and Luis Balart. *Sugar Busters! Quick and Easy Cookbook*. New York: Ballantine Books, 1999.

Cookbooks Available Through the Internet

The cookbooks are presented in alphabetical order by the author's name. They can be ordered through the indicated web site.

Laughlin, Brenda, and Kelly Nason. *Cooking Low Carb*.
Site name: C'est Bon Cookbooks
Site address: http://www.cest-bon.com/cookbooks.html

Railey, Brett. *The Skinny on Low Carb Cooking: Low Carb Wisdom From the Net*.
Site name: LCDP Low Carb Cookbook
Site address: http://lowcarbdieters.com/cookbook.htm

Internet Recipe Web Sites

These web sites contain recipes that can be printed or downloaded without charge. They are presented in alphabetical order by the site name. Site visitors post many of the recipes, and, therefore, many of the recipes are not kitchen-tested.

Mixed Recipe Web Sites

The following web sites are mixed in that they are not oriented to any one reduced carbohydrate plan.

Site name: alt.support.diet.low-carb
Site address: http://www.camacdonald.com/lc/lowcarbohydratecooking-recipes.htm

Site name: Carb Health
Site address: http://www.e-clipse.com

Site name: Carb Smart
Site address: http://www.carbsmart.com

Site name: Florida Lowcarb Corner
Site address: http://www.se.mediaone.net/~zibbler/LC_home.htm

Site name: ivillage.com
Site address: http://www.ivillage.com/diet/boards/

Site name: LivingSlim.com
Site address: http://www.livingslim.com

Site name: The Low Carb Cafe
Site address: http://www.lowcarbcafe.com

Site name: Low Carb Luxury
Site address: http://www.lowcarbluxury.com

Site name: The Low Carbohydrate Diets Information Center
Site address: http://people.delphi.com/elizjack/index.html

Site name: Low Carbohydrate Recipes
Site address: http://www.photopics.com/lowcarb.html

Site name: Lowcarb Cooking Cookbook
Site address: http://www.peavine.com/lowcarb/cookbook.html

Site name: Low-Carb Diet Information Clearinghouse
Site address: http://www.lowcarb.ca

Site name: LowCarbEating.com
Site address: http://lowcarbeating.com

Site name: Low-Carb Gourmet
Site address: http://www.lowcarbgourmet.com

Site name: Our Little (Low-Carbohydrate) Corner of the Internet
Site address: http://www.ourlittlecorner.com

Site name: Splenda.com
Site address: http://www.splenda.com

Site name: Thinner.com
Site address: http://www.thinner.com

Site name: 3 Fat Chicks on a Diet!
Site address: http://3fatchicks.com

Site name: Vegetarian Lowcarb
Site address: http://www.immuneweb.org/lowcarb

Atkins Diet Recipe Web Sites

Site name: Atkins & Low Carb Friends.com
Site address: http://atkinsfriends.com

Site name: Atkins Chat.com
Site address: http://www.atkinschat.com

Site name: The Atkins Diet Help.com
Site address: http://www.atkinsdiethelp.com

Site name: Everything Atkins
Site address: http://www7.addr.com/~atkinsdiet

Site name: Low Carb Lifestyles
Site address: http://www.bnatural.com/lowcarb/home.htm

Carbohydrate Addict's Diet Recipe Web Sites

Site name: Carbohydrate Addict's Network (official web
site of the Carbohydrate Addict's Program)
Site address: http://www.carbohydrateaddicts.com

Site name: Sugar Addict.com
Site address: http://www.sugaraddict.com

Paleolithic Diet Recipe Web Site

Site name: Paleo Food.com
Site address: http://www.panix.com/~paleodiet/list

Protein Power Diet Recipe Web Site

Site name: Protein Power (official web site of Protein Power)
Site address: http://www.eatprotein.com

Sugar Busters! Diet Recipe Web Site

Site name: Sugar Busters!.com (official web site of Sugar Busters!)
Site address: http://www.sugarbusters.com

The Zone Diet Recipe Web Sites

Site name: drsears.com (official web site of the Zone diet)
Site address: http://www.drsears.com

Site name: Zone Home
Site address: http://www.zonehome.com

Site name: Zone Perfect.com (official web site of the Zone diet)
Site address: http://zoneperfect.com

Commercial Web Sites

One of the great benefits of the Internet for reduced carbohydrate dieters is the easy availability of low carbohydrate foods, supplements, and products. In response to the growing demand for low carbohydrate products, many retailers have developed on-line stores that cater to the reduced carbohydrate dieter. Because of the popularity of these web sites, many of these products are making their way onto supermarket and retail outlet shelves. However, several popular low carbohydrate products are available only through the Internet.

Mixed Commercial Web Sites

The following on-line stores are not oriented to any one reduced carbohydrate plan.

Site name: a la Carb
Site address: alacarb.heyyoukids.com
Site features: Food, supplements, and products

Site name: Better Nutrition
Site address: http://www.deepdiscountnutrition.com
Site features: Food, supplements, and products

Site name: Carb Health
Site address: http://www.e-clipse.com
Site features: Books

Site name: Carb Smart
Site address: http://www.carbsmart.com
Site features: Books, food, products, and supplements

Site name: Diet Depot, Inc.
Site address: http://www.dietdepot.com
Site features: Food, supplements, and products

Site name: Expert Foods
Site address: http://members.tripod.com/~Expert_Foods
Site features: Food

Site name: Ketogenics, Inc.
Site address: http://www.ketogenics.com

Site features: Food and products

Site name: Life Services Supplements
Site address: http://www.lifeservices.com/catalog.htm
Site features: Supplements, books, and food

Site name: Low Carb Cafe
Site address: http://www.lowcarbcafe.com
Site features: Books

Site name: Low Carb Connoisseur
Site address: http://www.drugstore.com
Site features: Food, supplements, and products

Site name: Low Carb Dieter's Page
Site address: http://www.lowcarbdieters.com
Site features: Books, food, supplements, and products

Site name: Low Carb Living Market
Site address: http://www.lowcarbliving.com
Site features: Books and food

Site name: Low Carb Nexus
Site address: http://www.lowcarbnexus.com
Site features: Food, supplements, and products

Site name: Low Carb Outfitters
Site address: http://www.lowcarboutfitters.com
Site features: Books, food, supplements, and products

Site name: Lowcarb.com
Site address: http://www.lowcarb.com
Site features: Books, food, supplements, and products

Site name: LowCarbEating.com
Site address: http://lowcarbeating.com
Site features: Books, food, and products

Site name: LowCarbolicious!
Site address: http://www.lowcarbolicious.com
Site features: Pizza

Site name: Netrition.com
Site address: http://www5.netrition.com
Site features: Books, food, supplements, and products

Site name: Nutrition World
Site address: http://www.smartcart.com/nutworld/catalog
Site features: Books, food, supplements, and products

Site name: 1 Stop Sugarless Shop
Site address: http://www.sugarlessshop.com
Site features: Supplements and products

Site name: peakhealth.net
Site address: http://www.peakhealth.com
Site features: Food and supplements

Site name: Splenda.com
Site address: http://www.splenda.com
Site features: Splenda and products containing Splenda

Site name: Sugar Free Marketplace
Site address: http://www.sugarfreemarket.com
Site features: Atkins food, supplements, and products

Site name: Sugar Free Paradise
Site address: http://www.sugarfreeparadise.com

Site features: Sucralose and products containing sucralose

Site name: The Synergy Diet.com
Site address: http://www.synergydiet.com
Site features: Food, supplements, and products

Site name: Thinner.com
Site address: http://www.thinner.com
Site features: Books and Atkins products

Site name: Vitastorm.com
Site address: http://www.vitastorm.com
Site features: Books, food, supplements, and products

Site name: Yahoo! Low Carb Treats
Site address: http://store.yahoo.com/locarbn/index.html
Site features: Cookbook, magazine, food, supplements, and products

Atkins-Oriented Commercial Web Sites

Site name: Atkins & Low Carb Friends.com
Site address: http://atkinsfriends.com
Site features: Products

Site name: Atkins Center for Complementary Medicine
Site address: http://atkinscenter.com
Site features: Atkins books, foods, supplements, and products

Site name: The Atkins Diet Help.com
Site address: http://www.atkinsdiethelp.com
Site features: Books and supplements

Site name: drugstore.com
Site address: http://www.drugstore.com
Site features: Atkins food, supplements, and products

Site name: Everything Atkins
Site address: http://www7.addr.com/~atkinsdiet
Site features: Books

Carbohydrate Addict's Diet–Oriented Commercial Web Sites

Site name: Carbohydrate Addict's Network (official web site of the Carbohydrate Addict's Program)
Site address: http://www.carbohydrateaddicts.com
Site features: Carbohydrate Addict's books

Protein Power–Oriented Commercial Web Site

Site name: Protein Power (official web site of Protein Power)
Site address: http://www.eatprotein.com
Site features: Protein Power food, supplements, and products

Sugar Busters!–Oriented Commercial Web Site

Site name: Sugar Busters!.com (official site of Sugar Busters!)
Site address: http://www.sugarbusters.com
Site features: Sugar Busters! books and products

The Zone Diet–Oriented Commercial Web Sites

Site name: drsears.com (official site of the Zone diet)
Site address: http://www.drsears.com
Site features: Zone books, food, supplements, products, and services

Site name: Zone Home
Site address: http://www.zonehome.com
Site features: Zone books, products, and services

Site name: Zone Perfect.com (official site of the Zone Diet)
Site address: http://zoneperfect.com
Site features: Zone books, food, supplements, products, and services

Miscellaneous Resources

Book Review Web Sites

These web sites allow readers to post unbiased opinions of books. Readers can also rate a book on a scale of zero stars to five stars.

Site name: Amazon.com
Site address: http://www.amazon.com
Site features: Reduced carbohydrate diet book summaries and reviews

Site name: Barnes & Noble
Site address: http://www.bn.com
Site features: Reduced carbohydrate diet book summaries and reviews

Diabetes Resources

Drum, David, and Terry Zierenberg. *The Type 2 Diabetes Sourcebook: The Insulin Control Diet: Your Fat Can*

Make You Thin, second edition. Lowell, MA: Lowell House, 2000.

Site name: Diabetes
Site address: http://www.delphi.com/diabetes

Epilepsy Resources

Site name: Johns Hopkins Medicine, the Epilepsy Center, the Ketogenic Diet
Site address: http://www.neuro.jhmi.edu/Epilepsy/keto.html
Site features: Information about using ketogenic diets to control epileptic seizures

Site name: Ketogenic Diet at Packard Children's Hospital at Stanford University Medical Center
Site address: http://www.stanford.edu/group/ketodiet
Site features: Information exchange for healthcare providers using ketogenic diets to treat epilepsy

Glycemic Index Resources

Bahan, Deanie Comeaux. *Sugarfree New Orleans: A Cookbook Based on the Glycemic Index*. New Orleans: AFM Publishing, 1997.

Brand-Miller, Jennie; Kaye Foster-Powell; and Stephen Colagiuri. *The GI Factor: The Glycemic Index Solution*. Sydney, Australia: Hodder Headline, 1996.

Brand-Miller, Jennie; Thomas M.S. Wolever; Stephen Colagiuri; and Kaye Foster-Powell. *The Glucose Revolution: The Authoritative Guide to the Glycemic Index— the Groundbreaking Discovery*. New York: Marlowe & Company, 1996.

Site name: The Glycemic Index
Site address: http://www.cruzio.com/~mendosa/gi.htm
Site features: Information about glycemic index including links to other web sites, glycemic index databases, and food lists

Hypothyroidism Web Sites

Site name: American Thyroid Association
Site address: http://www.thyroid.org/index.htm
Site features: Hypothyroidism information and links

Site name: EndocrineWeb.com
Site address: http://www.endocrineweb.com/hypo1.html
Site features: Information on causes, symptoms, dangers, diagnosis, and treatment of hypothyroidism

Nutrition Counters

These nutrition counters are the most popular ones currently on the market. They are in alphabetical order according to the author's last name.

Atkins, Robert C. *Dr. Atkins' New Carbohydrate Gram Counter.* New York: M. Evans and Company, 1997.

Blonz, Edward R. *The Nutrition Doctor's A-to-Z Food Counter.* New York: Signet, 1999.

Eades, Michael R., and Mary Dan Eades. *The Protein Power LifePlan Gram Counter.* New York: Warner Books, 2000.

Havala, Suzanne. *The Vegetarian Food Guide and Nutrition Counter.* New York: Berkley Publishing, 1997.

Heller, Rachel F., and Richard F. Heller. *The Carbohydrate Addict's Calorie Counter.* New York: Signet, 2000.

Heller, Rachel F., and Richard F. Heller. *The Carbohydrate Addict's Carbohydrate Counter.* New York: Signet, 2000.

Heller, Rachel F., and Richard F. Heller. *The Carbohydrate Addict's Fat Counter.* New York: Signet, 2000.

Heller, Rachel F., and Richard F. Heller. *The Carbohydrate Addict's Gram Counter.* New York: Signet, 2000.

Natow, Annette B. *The Carbohydrate, Fiber, and Sugar Counter.* New York: Pocket Books, 1999.

Natow, Annette B. *The Eating Out Food Counter.* New York: Pocket Books, 1998.

Natow, Annette B. *The Fast Food Nutrition Counter.* New York: Simon & Schuster, 1994.

Natow, Annette B. *The Most Complete Food Counter.* New York: Pocket Books, 1999.

Netzer, Corinne T. *The Complete Book of Food Counts.* New York: Dell, 2000.

Sonberg, Lynn. *The Complete Nutrition Counter.* New York: Berkley, 1993.

Nutritional Analysis Web Sites

Site name: Mike's Calorie and Fat Gram Chart for 1000 Foods
Site address: http://www.ntwrks.com/~mikev/chart5a.htm
Site features: Nutritional count charts sorted by carbohydrate content

Site name: Stanford University Department of Pharmacy
Site address: http://www.stanford.edu/group/ketodiet/kctomeds.html
Site features: Description of carbohydrate content of selected medications

Site name: University of Illinois Nutritional Analysis Tool
Site address: http://www.ag.uiuc.edu/~food-lab/nat/mainnat.html
Site features: Nutritional analysis and nutritional counts of foods

Paleolithic Web Sites

Site name: The Healing Crow
Site address: http://www.healingcrow.com/dietsmain/paleo/paleo.html
Site features: Summary of the Paleolithic diet

Site name: The Paleolithic Diet Page
Site address: http://www.panix.com/~paleodiet
Site features: Extensive list of resources including books and web site links

Research Collections

Site name: Josh Yelon's Low Carb Medical Research
Site address: http://www.lowcarb.org/josh_yelon/lowcarb_med.html
Site features: Low carbohydrate medical research articles

Site name: Wilstar's Low-Carb Pavilion
Site address: http://wilstar.com/lowcarb/research.htm
Site features: Low carbohydrate medical research information

Yeast Overgrowth Web Sites

Site name: The Candida Page
Site address: http://www.panix.com/~candida
Site features: Extensive list of resources including books and web site links

Site name: The Yeast Connection (official web site of Dr. William Crook)
Site address: http://candida-yeast.com
Site features: Extensive information on yeast overgrowth including a questionnaire

Other Resources

McDonald, Lyle. *The Ketogenic Diet*. Kearney, NE: Morris Publishing, 1998. A presentation of the ketogenic diet as a benefit in bodybuilding.

Site name: Essential Fats.com
Site address: http://www.essentialfats.com
Site features: Extensive information on essential fatty acids from Dr. Edward N. Siguel, M.D.

Site name: The Ultimate Low Carb Resource
Site address: http://www.geocities.com/alabastercat/lowcarb.html
Site features: Low carbohydrate diet information

Site name: Wilstar's Low-Carb Pavilion
Site address: http://wilstar.com/lowcarb
Site features: Low carbohydrate food guidelines, hidden carbohydrate, supportive research, basic biochemistry, and food pyramid information

A Note From the Author

This book is all about the wonderful insights I have gathered from my fellow reduced carbohydrate dieters, and, in the spirit of low carbohydrate fellowship, I would love to hear from you, too. I am particularly interested in your comments about the information in this book that helps you lose weight and any personal experiences you have in applying this advice to your diet. I would also love to hear your ideas on how I can improve this book. Please feel free to forward an e-mail message to me at my personal e-mail address at lowcarbsuccess@aol.com. I am looking forward to hearing from you.

Index